3RD EDITION

Don Nutbeam | Elizabeth Harris | Marilyn Wise

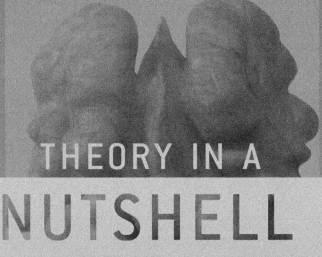

THEORY IN A
NUTSHELL

A practical guide to health promotion theories

The McGraw·Hill Companies

Sydney New York San Francisco Auckland
Bangkok Bogotá Caracas Hong Kong
Kuala Lumpur Lisbon London Madrid
Mexico City Milan New Delhi San Juan
Seoul Singapore Taipei Toronto

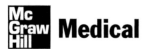
First published 1999
Second edition 2004
Reprinted 2014
Text © 2010 Don Nutbeam, Elizabeth Harris and Marilyn Wise
Illustrations and design © 2010 McGraw-Hill Australia Pty Ltd
Every effort has been made to trace and acknowledge copyrighted material. The authors and publishers tender their apologies should any infringement have occurred.

National Library of Australia Cataloguing-in-Publication Data

Author:	Nutbeam, Don
Title:	Theory in a nutshell: a practical guide to health promotion theories/ Don Nutbeam, Elizabeth Harris, Marilyn Wise
Edition:	3rd ed.
ISBN:	9780070278431 (pbk)
Notes:	Includes index, bibliography
Subjects:	Health promotion, health planning
Other Authors:	Harris, Elizabeth; Wise, Marilyn
Dewey Number:	613

Published in Australia by

McGraw-Hill Australia Pty Ltd
Level 2, 82 Waterloo Road, North Ryde NSW 2113

Publisher: Elizabeth Walton
Managing Editor: Kathryn Fairfax
Production Editor: Laura Carmody
Editorial Coordinator: Fiona Richardson
Art Director: Astred Hicks
Designer (cover and internals): Simon Rattray
Copyeditor: Nicole McKenzie
Proofreader: Terence Townsend
Indexer: Glenda Browne
Typeset in India by Mukesh Technologies
Printed in Australia by SOS Print + Media

contents

list of tables and figures

Chapter 4

Chapter 5

the purpose of this guide

Not all health promotion programs are equally successful in achieving their aims and objectives. Experience tells us that programs are most likely to be successful when the determinants of a health problem or issue are well understood, the needs and motivations of the target population are being addressed, and the context in which the program is being implemented has been taken into account. That is, when the program 'fits' the problem.

Although many health promotion projects and programs are developed and implemented without overt reference to theory, there is substantial evidence to suggest that the use of theory significantly improves the chance of success in achieving predetermined program objectives. The use of theory can help in the planning and delivery of programs in several ways. It can help us to:

- better understand the nature of the problem being addressed;
- describe and explain the needs and motivations of the target population;
- explain or make propositions concerning how to change health status, health-related behaviours and their determinants; and
- use evidence-informed methods and measures to monitor the problem and the program.

Theory therefore helps to achieve a better fit between problem and program.

This guide is intended to provide practitioners and students of health promotion with an overview of several of the most influential theories and models that have guided health promotion practice in the recent past, and that remain influential in the present.

For each theory discussed, an explanation of the main elements of the theory is provided, followed by a commentary on its relative strengths and weaknesses and some suggestions as to how it can be related to the 'real world'.

Through this guide, we hope to demonstrate that, when used prudently, theories can greatly enhance the effectiveness and sustainability of health promotion programs.

The use of theory can help to achieve a better fit between problem and program.

about the authors

Don Nutbeam is Vice-Chancellor of the University of Southampton, UK, and a Professor of Public Health. He was formerly Head of Public Health in the UK Department of Health.

Elizabeth Harris is Director of the Centre for Health Equity Training Research and Evaluation (CHETRE), which is part of UNSW Research Centre for Primary Health Care and Equity, University of New South Wales, Australia. Originally trained as a social worker and teacher, she has over 30 years' experience as a primary health care service provider and manager, population health researcher and teacher.

Marilyn Wise is Associate Professor of Healthy Public Policy at the Centre for Health Equity Training Research and Evaluation (CHETRE), which is part of the UNSW Research Centre for Primary Health Care and Equity, University of New South Wales, Australia. She has 20 years' experience as a health promotion practitioner, manager, researcher and teacher.

Acknowledgment
Several people have contributed to the development of the third edition of this guide. We would particularly like to acknowledge the contribution of Danielle Weber, who assisted with the review of the more recent literature.

the structure of this guide

This guide reflects the range of activities that are currently being undertaken by health promotion practitioners. It begins with an examination of those models that explain health behaviour and health behaviour change by focusing on characteristics of the individual. Four such theories/models that have been influential in health promotion practice are discussed:

- the health belief model;
- the themes of reasoned action and planned behaviour;
- the transtheoretical (stages of change) model; and
- the social cognitive theory.

What emerges from these overviews is that while these models contribute substantially to our understanding of individual behaviour, unless they also take into account the broader context in which the individual is living, many factors that influence health will remain unexplained.

It is now well recognised that the capacity and opportunities for individuals to bring about change to their health can be significantly affected by the characteristics and resources of the community in which they live, especially in addressing issues beyond the control of any one individual. This means that, as well as understanding theories of health that focus on the individual, we also need to understand theories that help explain how the capacity of communities can be strengthened, and how new ideas can best be introduced into communities. Correspondingly, theories of community mobilisation (as reflected in social planning, social action and community development) are discussed here, as is the 'diffusion of innovation' theory.

In order to raise awareness and engage individuals, groups and communities in taking action to promote health, a number of theories and models have been developed that provide guidelines on the ways in which health messages can be most effectively communicated and acted upon. Three of the most influential—health literacy (new to this edition), communication–behaviour change theory and social marketing theory—are discussed in this book. All three can provide very practical and effective guidance to people developing mass communication strategies. However, their impact will be limited if the relevant organisational structures do not support or facilitate the changes they seek to bring about.

Many organisational structures—also referred to as settings—can have both direct and indirect effects on people's health. Settings such as schools, worksites and recreational venues are places where people spend a great deal of time. Such settings directly influence health through the services and programs they provide to individuals and communities, and through the opportunities and constraints they place on individuals and health-related behaviours (e.g. facilities for physical activity, or restrictions on smoking). Less directly, such settings can influence health by providing access to social support or, negatively, by being a source of stress and conflict. They can also have indirect effects on health through, for example, planning regulations issued by councils or income support policies established by governments. In this context, this guide examines two categories of theories that help practitioners to understand how to influence change within organisations and enable them to work effectively together: theories of organisational change and a model for understanding intersectoral action.

Finally, this guide looks at the emerging field of healthy public policy and the models that are being developed to understand how policy can be influenced and changed to promote health. These include a framework for making healthy public policy; evidence-based policy making to promote health; and health impact assessment.

This third edition also includes revisions and updates to all sections. We have also attempted to introduce two important perspectives that this title has not considered before. Firstly, previous editions have not fully addressed the potential for differences in the effectiveness of interventions based on different theoretical approaches among different social groups. Certain theories may be more or less effective with the most socially disadvantaged in the population, and there is a risk that existing inequalities in health may be unintentionally exacerbated by inadequate attention to these effects. In truth, we have found relatively little evidence to guide our thinking on this issue. One perspective is that theories and models that support action directed to addressing the underlying social and economic determinants of health are more likely to have a positive impact on those who are most socially disadvantaged. Thus, those theories that support community building, organisational and policy change can be viewed as being more likely to have a positive impact on inequalities in health.

Secondly, we have not previously given significant attention to the potential application of the theories discussed in this guide to the improvement of mental health. As with the issue above, there is a similar risk that, without adequate attention, the application of different theories and models may have unintended negative effects on mental health. For example, it could be argued that the application of the health belief model, which depends on raising an individual's perception of risks to health, may have adverse consequences in the area of mental health. There are a number of emerging areas where health promotion practitioners are working, and where relevant theories and frameworks are emerging. Specifically, action to address health inequity and promotion of mental health can be expected to grow in the next few years. In the meantime, there is much to be learned from other disciplines, such as sociology, political science, psychology and human geography, which can inform action in the short term.

Table 1 Summary of theories and models presented in the guide

Approach	Theories or models
Theories and models that explain health behaviour and health behaviour change by focusing on the individual	Health belief model Theories of reasoned action and planned behaviour Transtheoretical (stages of change) model Social cognitive theory
Theories that explain change in terms of communities and communal action for health	Community mobilisation (planning, action, development) theory Diffusion of innovation theory
Theories that guide the use of communication strategies to bring about behavioural change to promote health	Health literacy model Communication–behaviour change theory Social marketing theory
Theories and models that explain how to influence change within organisations and create health-supportive organisational practices	Organisational change theories Intersectoral action models
Theories and models that explain the development and implementation of healthy public policy	A framework for making healthy public policy Evidence-based policy making to promote health Health impact assessment (HIA)

1

Theory

Most health promotion theories come from the behavioural and social sciences. They borrow from various disciplines such as psychology, sociology, management, consumer behaviour, marketing and the political sciences. Such diversity reflects the fact that health promotion practice is not only concerned with the behaviour of individuals but also with the ways in which society is organised and the policies and organisational structures that underpin social organisation.

Many of the theories commonly used in health promotion are not highly developed in the way suggested in the definition below, nor have they been rigorously tested when compared, for example, with theory in the physical sciences. Many of the theories included in this book could be better described as theoretical frameworks or models.

Health promotion theories and models can help to bind together our observations and ideas, and make sense of them.

1.1 What is a theory?

A fully developed theory explains:

- the **major factors that influence the phenomenon of interest**—for example, those factors that explain why some people are regularly active and others are not;
- the **relationship between these factors**—for example, the relationship between knowledge, beliefs, social norms and behaviours (such as physical activity); and
- the **conditions under which these relationships do or do not occur**, or the *how*, *when* and *why* of hypothesised relationships—for example, the time, place and circumstances that, predictably, lead to a person being either active or inactive.

One commonly used definition of a theory is:

> Systematically organised knowledge applicable in a relatively wide variety of circumstances devised to analyse, predict, or otherwise explain the nature or behaviour of a specified set of phenomena that could be used as the basis for action (Van Ryn & Heany 1992).

1.2   The use of theory

The potential for theory to guide the development of health promotion interventions is substantial. Several different planning models are used by health promotion practitioners, among the best known being the precede–proceed model developed by Green & Kreuter (2005). Several variations of this approach have also been produced (see the references at the end of this chapter for more information).

Each of these planning models follows a structured sequence, including planning, implementation and evaluation stages. Reference to different theories can guide and inform practitioners at each of these stages.

Figure 1 below presents a health promotion planning cycle, indicating the various steps involved in the planning, implementation and evaluation of a health promotion program. These steps are discussed in detail opposite.

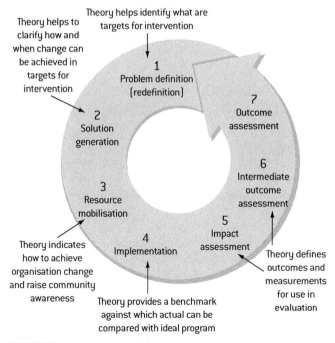

Figure 1 Health promotion planning and evaluation cycle

Defining the problem

Identifying the parameters of the health problem to be addressed may involve drawing on a wide range of epidemiological and demographic information, as well as on information from the behavioural and social sciences and knowledge of community needs and priorities. Here, different theories can help us to identify *what* should be the focus of the intervention.

Specifically, theory can inform our choice of which elements of the health problem we should consider as the focus of the intervention. For example, the health belief model and the theory of reasoned action help to identify the individual characteristics, beliefs and values that are associated with different health behaviours and that may be possible to change. Organisational change theory helps to identify the key elements of organisations that may need to be changed and that may be possible to change.

Planning a solution

The second step in the planning cycle is the analysis of potential solutions, leading to the development of a program plan which specifies the objectives and strategies to be employed, as well as the sequence of activities that will be used to achieve them. Theory is at its most useful here in providing guidance on *how* and *when* change might be achieved in the target population, organisation or policy. It may also offer ideas that would not otherwise have occurred to us.

Different theories can help us to understand what methods we can use as the focus of our interventions, specifically by improving our understanding of the processes by which changes occur in the target variables (i.e. people, organisations or policies), and by clarifying the most effective means of achieving change in these target variables. For example, the social cognitive theory helps to explain the relationship between personal observation and experience, social norms and the influence of external environments, and the effects of these factors on individual behaviour. The insights into these relationships that are provided by the social cognitive theory can help in the design of a program, for instance by indicating how changes to the environment or to social norms can affect health behaviour.

Thus, those theories that explain and predict individual and group health behaviour and organisational practice, as well as those that identify methods for changing these determinants of health behaviour and organisational practice, are worthy of close consideration in this phase of planning.

Some theories also inform decisions on the timing and sequencing of our interventions in order to achieve maximum effects. For example, the transtheoretical (stages of change) model and the diffusion of innovation theory provide guidance on the timing and sequence of activities involving individuals and communities.

Mobilising resources

Once a program plan has been developed, the first step in the implementation stage is usually directed towards generating public and political interest in the program, mobilising resources for program implementation and building capacity in partner organisations through which the program will operate (such as schools, worksites or local governments). Models of intersectoral action, which help us understand how to build partnerships, and organisational change theory, which indicates how to influence organisational policy and procedures, are particularly useful here, as is communication–behaviour change theory, which can guide the development of media-based awareness-raising activities.

Implementing the program

The implementation of a program may involve multiple strategies, such as education and advocacy. Here, the key elements of theory can provide a benchmark against which the actual selection of methods and sequencing of an intervention can be considered in relation to the theoretically ideal implementation of a program.

In this way, the use of theory helps us to explain success or failure in different programs, particularly by highlighting the possible effects of any differences between what was planned and what actually occurred in the implementation of the program. It can also assist us in identifying the key elements of a program which can form the basis of future successful programs.

Evaluating the program

Health promotion interventions can be expected to have different levels of impact and different effects over time. Impact evaluation represents the first level of outcome evaluation of a program. The adoption of theory in the planning of programs can provide guidance on the measures that can be used to assess the success of programs. For example, where theory suggests that the target of an intervention is to achieve changes in knowledge and self-efficacy, or changes in social norms or organisational practices, measurement of these changes becomes the first point of evaluation. Such measures are often referred to as 'health promotion outcomes'.

Intermediate outcome assessment is the next level of evaluation. Theory can also be used to predict the intermediate health outcomes that are sought from an intervention. Usually these are considered in terms of modification of individual behaviour or modifications to social, economic and environmental conditions that determine health or influence behaviour. Several theories, such as the health belief model and the social cognitive theory, predict that changes to health promotion outcomes will lead to changes in health behaviour.

Health outcome assessment refers to the end-point outcomes of an intervention in terms of change in physical or mental health status, in quality of life, or in improved equity of health within populations. Definitions of these final outcomes will be based on theoretically predicted relationships between changes in the determinants of risk (intermediate health outcomes) and final health outcomes.

Figure 1 (page 2) indicates that each of the steps taken in the evaluation stage leads back to a redefinition of the prioritised problems and solutions, hence the concept of a cycle of planning and evaluation.

Table 2 below summarises the tasks involved and the potential uses of theory to support each step in the planning, implementation and evaluation stages of a health promotion program.

Table 2 Use of theory in program planning, implementation and evaluation

Step	Task	Potential use of theory
Defining the problem	Clarify major health issues for a defined population, and prioritise these in terms of the potential for effective intervention	Guidance on what should be the target elements of the intervention, e.g. individual beliefs, social norms or organisational practices
Planning a solution	Develop a program plan that specifies objectives, strategies and the sequence of activities to be undertaken	Guidance on how, when and where change can be achieved in the target elements of the program
Mobilising resources	Generate public and political support, build the capacity of partner organisations and secure resources	Guidance on how to build partnerships, raise public awareness and foster organisational development
Implementing the program	Implement the program as planned, using multiple strategies as appropriate to the program objectives	Guidance on a benchmark against which the actual implementation can be considered in relation to the theoretical ideal
Evaluating the program	Assess the effects and outcomes of the program with reference to the program objectives	Guidance on outcomes and measurements that can be used at each level of evaluation

1.3   A single theory or multiple theories?

Theories are not static pronouncements that can be applied to all issues under all circumstances. Some of the theories used in health promotion have been extensively refined and developed in the light of experience. The range and focus of theories available has also expanded over the past two decades, from a focus purely on the modification of individual behaviour to a recognition of the need to influence and change a broad range of social, economic and environmental factors that influence health alongside individual behavioural choices.

Thus, contemporary health promotion operates at several different levels, namely:

- the individual;
- the community;
- the organisation; and
- public policy and practice.

Choosing the right approach will depend on the nature of the problem, its determinants and the opportunities for action.

Programs that operate at multiple levels, such as those that draw on combinations of the strategies described in the Ottawa Charter for Health Promotion, are the most likely to address the range of determinants of health problems in populations, and thereby have the greatest effect.

For example, a program to improve uptake of immunisation will generally be more effective if it involves a combination of interventions. These might include:

- education to inform and motivate individual parents to immunise their children;
- facilitation of community debate to change perceptions about the safety and convenience of immunisation;
- changes to organisational practice to improve notification systems;
- provision of more conveniently located clinics; and
- financial incentives for parents and health practitioners.

Successful implementation of such a program of activity might draw on several theories. For example, educational programs could make use of the health belief model to shape messages about the threat of vaccine-preventable diseases and the benefits of immunisation; community debate could be stimulated using social marketing methods; organisational change theory could help to improve clinic practices; and so on. It follows that no single theory dominates health promotion practice, and nor could it, given the range of health problems and their determinants, the diversity of populations and settings, and the differences in available resources, skills and opportunities for action among practitioners.

Depending on the level of intervention (individual, group or organisation) and the type of change being aimed for (simple, one-off behaviour, complex behaviour, organisational or policy change), different theories will have greater relevance and better 'fit' the problem.

None of the theories or models presented in this book can simply be adopted as the answer to all problems. Most often, we benefit by drawing on more than one of the theories presented here to match the multiple levels of the program response being aimed for.

In many cases it will be possible and appropriate to combine different models and theories to achieve goals across the spectrum of health promotion actions.

To be useful and relevant, the different theories and models need to be readily understood and genuinely capable of application to a wide variety of real-life conditions of practice. Although social psychologist Kurt Lewin declared that 'there is nothing so practical as a good theory' (Hunt 1987), many of us remain somewhat sceptical of the capacity of intervention theories to provide the guidance necessary to develop an effective intervention in a complex environment.

Karen Glanz (2008) offers a commonsense summary of how to judge whether a theory or combination of theories is a good fit with the problem being addressed. She says it is a good fit if it is:

■ logical;
■ consistent with everyday observations;
■ similar to those used in previous successful programs you have read or heard about; and
■ supported by past research in the area or related areas.

Ultimately, theories and models are simplified representations of reality; they can never include or explain all of the complexities of individual, social or organisational behaviours. However, while the use of theory alone does not guarantee effective programs, the use of theory in the planning, execution and evaluation of programs will enhance the chance of success.

One of the greatest challenges for practitioners is to identify how to best achieve a fit between the issues of interest and the established theories or models that could improve the effectiveness of a program or intervention. This book is intended to assist you in meeting this challenge.

References

Glanz K, Rimer BK & Viswanath K (Eds) 2008, *Health behavior and health education: theory, research and practice*, 4th edn, Jossey-Bass, San Francisco, CA.

Green LW & Kreuter MW 2005, *Health promotion planning: an educational and ecological approach*, 4th edn, McGraw-Hill, New York, NY.

Hunt DE 1987, *Beginning with ourselves: in practice, theory and human affairs*, Brookline Books, Cambridge, MA, p. 4.

Van Ryn M & Heany CA 1992, 'What's the use of theory?', *Health Education Quarterly*, vol. 19, no. 3, pp. 315–330.

World Health Organization (WHO) 1986, *Ottawa Charter for Health Promotion*, WHO, Geneva. Available online at http://www.who.int/healthpromotion/conferences/previous/ottawa/en/.

Further reading

1.2 The use of theory

Nutbeam D & Bauman A 2006, *Evaluation in a nutshell: a practical guide to the evaluation of health promotion programs*, McGraw-Hill, Sydney.

2

Theories which explain health behaviour and health behaviour change by focusing on individual characteristics

One of the major roots of contemporary health promotion can be found in the application of health psychology to bring about health behaviour change. Evidence for this can be seen in the phenomenal growth of the discipline of health psychology and in the evolution of the concept of behavioural medicine. The discipline of health psychology has had a particularly significant influence in the United States, where for several decades researchers have sought to explain, predict and change health behaviour by means of the development and application of theories and models evolving from the disciplines of psychology and social psychology. In this chapter we discuss three of the most enduring and influential models of this kind.

2.1 The health belief model

The health belief model is one of the longest established theoretical models designed to explain health behaviour by better understanding individuals' beliefs about health. It was originally advanced to explain why individuals participate in public health screening and immunisation programs, and has since been developed for application to other types of health behaviour.

At its core, this model suggests that the likelihood of an individual taking action related to a given health problem is based on the interaction between four different types of belief. Figure 2 overleaf summarises these four elements. The model predicts that individuals will take action to protect or promote health if:

- they perceive themselves to be susceptible to a condition or problem;
- they believe it would have potentially serious consequences;
- they believe a course of action is available that will reduce their susceptibility or minimise the consequences; and
- they believe that the benefits of taking action outweigh the costs or barriers.

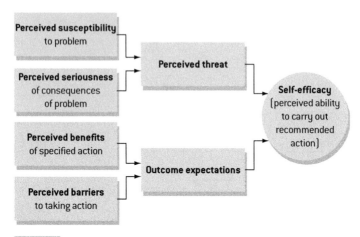

Figure 2 Health belief model: major components and linkages

Later refinements have acknowledged important modifying factors, particularly those associated with personal characteristics and social circumstances, as well as the influence of more immediate cues for action, such as media publicity and personal experience. Added to this analysis is the concept of self-efficacy—that is, the belief in one's own ability to successfully perform a behaviour—as a further factor influencing the strength of the model in predicting behaviour change.

Thus, for example, if we consider the application of this model to the prevention of HIV infection, in order to adopt behaviours that minimise their risk of infection, individuals would need to:

- believe that they are at risk of HIV infection;
- believe that the consequences of infection would be serious;
- receive cues for action that may trigger a response (such as targeted media publicity);
- believe that risk-minimisation practices (such as safe sex or abstinence) will greatly reduce the risk of infection;
- believe that the benefits of taking action to reduce risk outweigh the potential costs and barriers (such as reduced enjoyment and negative reactions of their partner and/or the community); and
- believe in their ability to take effective action (self-efficacy), such as by following safe sex practices.

Although it was not always consciously done, many of the early public-education campaigns concerning HIV/AIDS prevention took this approach. Initially this was done by seeking to persuade people that they were at risk, and by emphasising the deadly nature of AIDS. Later, as the epidemic developed, public-education campaigns focused more on the efficacy of safe sex (particularly the use of condoms) in minimising the risk of infection, and on improving people's confidence to use condoms.

Successive 1974 and 1984 reviews of findings from interventions using the health belief model provided reasonably consistent evidence to support the usefulness of the model in predicting why individuals adopted (or failed to adopt) different health behaviours. In the 25 years since the publication of the more recent review, the model has been widely adopted as a planning tool for health education programs intended to promote greater compliance with preventive health behaviours and healthcare recommendations.

Subsequent reviews (in 1992) and practical application have provided rather more mixed evidence of success, but have helped to refine our understanding of the best application of the model and have led to some tailored variations to the model being developed, for example, to support mammography screening uptake. Through this continuous testing, overcoming perceived barriers to successful action, along with providing cues for action, have been identified as the most important elements of the model. Perceived susceptibility and perceived benefits were also recognised as important.

In a 1984 review of the model, the authors pointed to the limitations of the model in predicting and explaining health behaviour:

> The health belief model is a psychosocial model; as such it is limited to accounting for as much of the variance in an individual's health behaviour as can be explained by their attitudes and beliefs. It is clear that other forces influence health actions as well (Janz & Becker 1984).

These 'other forces' include social, economic and environmental conditions, which significantly shape the barriers to action that are fundamental to the model. For example, limited access to healthcare services and/or resources can, of course, greatly impede effective health actions, and will in turn influence the individual's perceptions of barriers and benefits that are integral to the model.

If we go back to the example of the HIV/AIDS public-education campaigns, some of the limitations of the health belief model become apparent. The lack of accessible sexually transmissible diseases services, the cost or lack of availability of condoms, and pressures on groups such as sex workers to act in unsafe ways in order to keep customers, can all work against people adopting behaviours that they know will reduce their risk of infection. Individual behaviour and the beliefs that influence it therefore need to be seen in this wider context.

Commentary

The health belief model has been found to be most useful when applied to those behaviours for which it was originally developed, particularly traditional preventive health behaviours such as screening and immunisation. It has been less useful in guiding interventions to address more long-term, complex and socially determined behaviours, such as alcohol, tobacco and other drug use. Because the model takes little account of social, economic and environmental influences on behaviour, it is also limited in the extent to which it might be used to address socially determined inequalities in health.

The model's main benefit is the relatively simple way in which it illustrates the importance of individual beliefs about health and about the relative costs and benefits of actions designed to protect or improve health. Three decades of research have indicated that promoting change in those beliefs can lead to changes in health behaviour that contribute to improved health status. Changes in knowledge and beliefs will almost always form part of a comprehensive health promotion program, and the health belief model provides an essential reference point in the development of messages to improve knowledge and change beliefs, especially those designed for use in the media.

2.2 The theories of reasoned action and planned behaviour

The theory of reasoned action was developed by Ajzen and Fishbein (1980) to explain human behaviour that is under 'voluntary' control. A major assumption underlying the theory is that people are usually rational and will make predictable decisions in well-defined circumstances. This model is predicated on the assumption that intention to act is the most immediate determinant of behaviour, and that all other factors influencing behaviour will be mediated through behavioural intention.

The upper part of Figure 3 below shows how behavioural intentions are thought to be influenced by attitudes towards behaviours and subjective norms. Attitudes, in this case, are determined by the belief that a desired outcome will occur if a particular behaviour is followed, and that the outcome will be beneficial to health (this concept is similar to that of perceived benefits

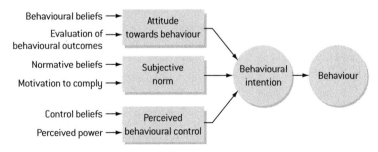

Figure 3 Theory of planned behaviour: major components and linkages

and barriers in the health belief model). This part of the figure summarises Ajzen and Fishbein's original theory of reasoned action (1980).

Subjective norms in this case relate to a person's beliefs about what other people think he or she should do (normative beliefs), and to the person's motivation to comply with those other people's wishes. These social influences vary in strength, depending on the degree to which the individual values social approval by a particular group. For example, if an individual who smokes feels that most people do not smoke and that most of his or her valued friends and colleagues want him or her to quit, then it is most likely that the person would consider that there is a norm that favours quitting smoking.

Intentions to act are thus jointly determined by attitudes and subjective norms. Put simply, the theory predicts that a person is most likely to intend to adopt, maintain or change a behaviour if that person believes that the behaviour will benefit their health, believes that the behaviour is socially desirable and feels social pressure to behave in that way. According to the theory, if these beliefs and social pressures are strong enough, this intention to behave will subsequently be transferred into behaviour. By influencing beliefs and exerting social pressure, behaviours can therefore be changed or maintained.

Ajzen and Fishbein take this analysis a step further by indicating that it is the short-term consequences of behaviours that are the most powerful in predicting attitudes towards behaviour, and that subjective norms are most affected by significant others. These significant others might include, for example, a person's valued peers, as well as media and sports celebrities who are seen as role models.

Ajzen and others have developed this theory further and have added perceived behavioural control as a third influence on behavioural intentions. This recognises that a person's intentions will become significantly greater if they feel they have greater personal control over a behaviour— a concept closely allied to self-efficacy—and that this is also mediated by their perceived power in relation to a given situation. In making this adjustment Ajzen recognised that there are many factors beyond the immediate control of individuals that shape their ability to behave in a desired way. As a consequence, Ajzen (1985) proposed changing the theory's name from the 'theory of reasoned action' to the 'theory of planned behaviour'.

This theory can be very useful in identifying what information you might need to collect from a target group before developing a program. It highlights the need to understand the beliefs of the group about the issue, about who they see as affecting these beliefs and their behaviour, and about what they perceive as barriers to taking actions that might promote their health.

For example, in developing a heart health education program in a minority ethnic community, it would be important to understand what the members of this target group believe are the causes of heart disease, and what actions they feel they can confidently take to reduce their risk. It would also be important to identify the significant others who shape the decisions that could reduce the risk of heart disease. For example, if the program was trying to change people's eating patterns, it might be the eldest woman in the household or the eldest son who has most influence over the family's diet.

Ajzen and Fishbein's original model was widely applied to the development of programs to reduce the uptake of smoking among youth during the 1980s. These programs recognised that information on the consequences of smoking should emphasise the short-term negative consequences (such as effects on appearance and financial cost), as opposed to the long-term negative consequences (such as lung cancer and heart disease). Such programs also recognised the role of significant others in shaping decisions to smoke, by using peer leaders in smoking education programs and recruiting acknowledged role models for young people. More recently this theory has been applied to the development of programs to reduce the transmission of HIV and other sexually transmitted diseases.

Commentary

The results of the smoking education programs referred to above were weaker than expected, resulting in the modifications to the theory described above. Subsequent applications of the model have demonstrated its usefulness in identifying factors that influence health behaviour and that may be targets for intervention.

Past failures of programs based on the theory of reasoned action have highlighted not only the difficulty of translating models that predict behaviour change into successful health promotion interventions, but also the dangers of choosing to focus on just a few elements in a complex model. The model is most successfully applied when all elements are considered. Its proponents stress the importance of conducting in-depth interviews to identify the most important beliefs that are relevant to the behaviour concerned. As with the health belief model, the theory of reasoned action provides valuable insight into key factors that influence behaviour, and provides a strong indication of the importance of perceived social norms and of an understanding of short-term consequences in shaping health behaviour.

2.3   The transtheoretical (stages of change) model

The transtheoretical (stages of change) model was developed by Prochaska and DiClemente to describe and explain the different stages of change that appear to be common to most behaviour change processes. The model has two basic dimensions, describing both the *stages of change* and the *processes of change* relevant to the different stages. The model is based on the premise that behaviour change is a process rather than an event, and that individuals have varying levels of motivation or readiness to change. It identifies five basic stages of change:

- **precontemplation**—this describes individuals who are not even considering changing their behaviour, as well as those who are consciously intending not to change;
- **contemplation**—the stage at which a person considers making a change to a specific behaviour;
- **determination** (or preparation)—the stage at which a person makes a serious commitment to change;
- **action**—the stage at which behaviour change is initiated; and,
- **maintenance**—the stage of sustaining the change, and of the achievement of predictable health gains. **Relapse** may also be the fifth stage.

A sixth stage—**termination**—has also been identified as being appropriate to some behaviours, especially addictive behaviours. This represents a stage at which individuals have no temptation and high self-efficacy in relation to the changed behaviour, as though they had never acquired the habit (such as smoking) in the first place.

People appear to move in a predictable way through these stages, although some move more quickly than others, and some get 'stuck' at a particular stage. A person's confidence in their ability to change and to overcome perceived barriers, and 'decisional balance' (a person's relative weighting of the pros and cons of making a change) are among the factors identified as influencing progression between stages.

This model is circular rather than linear, as people can enter or exit at any point, and it applies equally to people who self-initiate change and those who respond to external stimuli such as advice from health professionals or health campaigns.

This model has application at both the individual and the broader program level. For example, for health practitioners this model provides a useful way of thinking about the advice that they give their patients, and may help to reduce the frustration they feel when their advice is not taken. The model provides a way of establishing whether their patient wants to change, assists in identifying barriers to change, and recognises that relapsing is a common problem in any change process (see Table 3 overleaf).

From a program planning perspective, this model is particularly useful in indicating how the different processes of change can influence how programs or activities should be staged. Prochaska et al. (2008) have identified several processes of change that are consistently useful in supporting movement between stages. These processes are more or less applicable at the various stages of change. For example, consciousness raising may be most useful among people at the precontemplation stage who may not be aware of the

Table 3 Use of the transtheoretical model by health practitioners to promote weight control among patients

Stage of change	Process of change	Action
Precontemplation	Consciousness raising	Discuss with the patient the health problems associated with being overweight and the feasibility of weight loss
Contemplation	Recognition of the benefits of change	Discuss with the patient the potential benefits to them of the proposed change (illustrate what success would mean)
Determination	Identification of barriers	Assist patient in identifying potential barriers they may face and how these can be addressed; emphasise the relative benefits to influence decisional balance
Action	Program of change	Develop a plan for weight loss with the patient that supports the development of self-efficacy and provides mechanisms for feedback
Maintenance	Follow-up and continuing support	Organise routine follow-ups and discuss with the patient the likelihood of relapse

threat to health that their behaviour poses, whereas communication of the benefits of change and illustration of the success of others in changing health behaviour may be most important for those at the contemplation stage. Once the change process has been initiated—at the action stage—social support and stimulus control (such as avoiding certain situations or having environmental supports in place) become important.

More recently, DiClemente (2005) has emphasised that the model has a third dimension, namely, the *context* of change. He stresses that the internal and external environment that surrounds the targeted health behaviour change makes a significant contribution to the process of change and to the movement or lack of movement through the stages of change. He makes the point that if a person works in an environment where it is difficult to smoke and difficult to make healthy food choices, then it will be easier for that person to quit smoking and harder for them to make healthy food choices.

By matching the stages of behavioural change with specific processes, this model specifies how interventions can be organised for different populations with different needs and different circumstances. It provides important advice on the need to research the characteristics of the target population;

the need not to assume that all people are at the same stage; and the need to organise interventions sequentially to address the different stages as they are encountered.

Commentary

The transtheoretical model has quickly become an important reference point in health interventions on a range of issues, including smoking cessation, physical activity, weight control and the use of preventive services such as mammography screening. Apart from the obvious advantage in health promotion of focusing on the change process, this model is important in that it emphasises the range of needs for intervention in any given population, the changing needs of different populations, and the need for sequencing of interventions to match the different stages of change. It illustrates the importance of tailoring programs to the real needs and circumstances of individuals, rather than assuming an intervention will be equally applicable to all.

A 2005 review of findings from health behaviour interventions using the transtheoretical model (Bridle et al.) found only limited evidence of effectiveness from interventions of 'highly variable quality'. The model has been criticised for failing to account for the full complexity of behavioural change processes. Although it has been proposed as a model that serves as an umbrella for other theories that guide health promotion practice, its strong roots in behavioural psychology and primary application in clinical settings with individuals makes this assessment somewhat optimistic. It may be best considered as a useful approach to defining needs and structuring interventions to improve the health of individuals or groups.

2.4   Social cognitive theory

Social cognitive theory is one of the most widely applied theories in health promotion because it addresses both the underlying determinants of health behaviour and methods of promoting change. Social cognitive theory has evolved with input from several researchers over the past 50 years but, in terms of its application to health promotion, the most influential writer has been Albert Bandura.

Social cognitive theory was built on an understanding of the interaction that occurs between an individual and their environment. Early psychosocial research tended to focus on the way in which environment shapes behaviour by making it more or less rewarding to behave in particular ways. For example, if a workplace has no regulations on where people are allowed to smoke, it is easy for employees to be smokers. If regulations are in place it is more difficult, and as a consequence most smokers will smoke less and will find such an environment more supportive for quitting.

Social cognitive theory indicates that the relationship between people and their environment is more subtle and complex. For example, in circumstances where a significant number of people are non-smokers and are assertive about their desire to restrict smoking in their environment, even without formal regulations, it becomes far less rewarding for individuals to smoke. They are then likely to modify their behaviour. In this case the non-smokers have influenced the smokers' perception of the environment (referred to in the theory as 'situation') through social influence.

Bandura refers to this principle as 'reciprocal determinism'. It describes the way in which an individual, their environment and their behaviour continuously interact and influence each other. An understanding of this interaction and of the way in which the modification of social norms can affect behaviour offers an important insight into how behaviour can be modified through health promotion interventions. For example, seeking to modify social norms regarding smoking has been shown to be a powerful way of promoting cessation among adults.

Added to this basic understanding of the relationship between behaviour and the environment, Bandura also determined that a range of personal cognitive factors form a third part to this relationship, affecting and being affected by specific behaviours and environments. Of these cognitions, three are particularly important. The first is the capacity to learn by observing both the behaviour of others and the rewards received for different behaviours (observational learning). For example, some young women may observe behaviours (such as smoking) by people whom they regard as sophisticated and attractive (role models). If they observe and value the rewards that they associate with smoking, such as sexual attractiveness or a desirable self-image, then they are more likely to smoke themselves—their expectancies in relation to smoking are positive. Such an understanding further reinforces the importance of taking into account peer influences and social norms on health behaviour, and of the potential use of role models in influencing social norms.

The second important cognition is the capacity to anticipate and place value on the outcomes of different behaviour patterns (referred to as 'expectations'). For example, if you believe that smoking will help you to lose weight and you place great value on losing weight, then you are more likely to take up or to continue smoking. This highlights the importance of understanding the personal beliefs and motivations underlying different behaviours, and the need to emphasise the short-term and tangible benefits or negative effects of behaviours. For example, young people have been shown to respond far more negatively to the short-term effects of smoking (bad breath, smelly clothes) than to any long-term threat posed to their health by lung cancer or heart disease.

Thirdly, Bandura's work (1997) developed the concept of self-efficacy (belief in one's own ability to successfully perform a behaviour). According to

Bandura, self-efficacy is the most important prerequisite for behaviour change, and will affect how much effort is put into a task and the outcome of that task. The promotion of self-efficacy is thus an important task in the achievement of behaviour change. Bandura proposed that both observational learning and participatory learning (such as by supervised practice and repetition) lead to the development of the knowledge and skills necessary for behaviour change (behavioural capability) and are powerful tools in building self-confidence and self-efficacy. In later refinements to this fundamental structure, Bandura described the importance of self-regulation—the capacity to endure short-term negative outcomes in pursuit of a long-term goal. He highlights the importance of goal setting and feedback in relation to behaviour change, as well as social support in maintaining change.

As is the case in the interaction between behaviour and the environment, the three-way relationship between these personal characteristics, behaviour and the environment is reciprocal and dynamic. For example, a young woman who is quitting smoking may be very confident (high self-efficacy) about her ability to abstain at work where smoking is banned and where none of her workmates smoke, but she may be less confident when she goes out with her friends who are heavy smokers. Thus, self-efficacy is both behaviour-specific and situation-specific (environment-specific).

This explicit acknowledgment of the dynamic and reciprocal relationship between an individual, their behaviour and the environment avoids overly simple solutions to health problems that focus on behaviour in isolation from the social environment. An understanding of the characteristics of the person assists in the creation of educational interventions to alter the knowledge, understanding, beliefs and skills that affect observational learning, outcome expectations and self-efficacy. Such interventions are intended to improve the capacity of an individual to behave in a desired way. Understanding the way in which the physical and social environments act to provide incentives or disincentives for different behaviours points to ways of constructing interventions to modify the environment to further support healthy behaviours, and provides opportunities to change. Recognition that the importance of factors relating to the person and the environment will vary with different behaviours adds further depth to the development of an intervention.

Commentary

Taken as a whole, social cognitive theory provides a comprehensive theoretical basis for health promotion programs. It recognises the fundamental importance of individual beliefs, values and self-confidence in determining health behaviour. It also explicitly identifies the importance of social norms and cues (social modelling) and environmental influences on health behaviour, and the continuous interaction between these variables. Social cognitive theory provides practical direction on how to modify these influences. In this sense it provides an important bridge between this section of the book and the sections that follow on community mobilisation, organisational change and public policy development.

This model also suggests a role for the health practitioner which may be less overtly interventionist than those implied by the models described earlier. The health worker becomes a 'change agent', facilitating change through modification of the social environment and development of self-efficacy in ways that enable individuals to act to improve their health.

It also assists in understanding the multiple levels at which a health promotion program may need to work. For example, in trying to reduce the number of young women who take up smoking, it may be as important to address the issue of body image as it is to provide information on the short- and long-term consequences of smoking. The influence of this model can be seen in the large number of health promotion interventions that combine educational programs with modification of the social and physical environments.

2.5   Summary

This overview of theories that explain health behaviour and health behaviour change by focusing on characteristics of the individual provides important guidance on the major elements of health promotion programs. Taken together, the models described above emphasise:

- the importance of knowledge and beliefs about health. All of the theories and models presented in this chapter imply a central role for health education and refer to individual knowledge about health. They emphasise the importance of personalising health information and stressing the short-term consequences of behaviours so that communication is more immediately relevant to individuals;
- the importance of self-efficacy, or the belief in one's own ability to successfully perform a behaviour. The development of the personal skills and self-confidence that create self-efficacy, through personal observation, supervised practice and repetition, is central to success in each of the models presented;
- the importance of perceived social norms and social influences, relating to the value an individual places on social approval or acceptance by various social groups. The influence of social role models, family and peer groups is emphasised here;

- the importance of recognising that individuals within a population may be at different stages of change at any one time;
- the limitations of psychosocial theories that do not adequately take into account those socioeconomic and environmental conditions that significantly shape access to services and resources; and
- the importance of shaping or changing the environment or people's perception of the environment as an important element of health promotion programs.

References

Ajzen I 1991, 'The theory of planned behaviour', *Organisational behaviour and human decision processes*, vol. 50, pp. 179–211.

Ajzen I 1985, 'From intentions to actions: a theory of planned behavior', in J Kuhl & J Beckmann (Eds), *Action control: from cognition to behavior*, Springer-Verlag, New York.

Ajzen I & Fishbein M 1980, *Understanding attitudes and predicting social behavior*, Prentice-Hall, Englewood Cliffs, NJ.

Bridle C, Reisma R & Pattenden J et al. 2005, 'Systematic review of the effectiveness of health behaviour interventions based on the transtheoretical model', *Psychology and Health*, vol. 20, no. 3, pp. 283–301.

DiClemente CC 2005, 'Conceptual models and applied research: the ongoing contribution of the transtheoretical model', *Journal of Addictions Nursing*, vol. 16, pp. 5–12.

Janz NK & Becker MH 1984, 'The health belief model: a decade later', *Health Education Quarterly*, vol. 1, pp. 1–47.

Prochaska JO, Redding CA & Evers KE 2008, 'The transtheoretical model and stages of change', in K Glanz, BK Rimer & K Viswanath (Eds), *Health behavior and health education: theory, research and practice*, 4th edn, Jossey-Bass, San Francisco, CA.

Further reading 2.1

Champion VL & Skinner CS 2008, 'The health belief model', in K Glanz, BK Rimer & K Viswanath (Eds), *Health behavior and health education: theory, research and practice*, 4th edn, Jossey-Bass, San Francisco, CA.

Harrison JA et al. 1992, 'A meta-analysis of studies of the health belief model', *Health Education Research*, vol. 7, no. 1, pp. 107–116.

Further reading 2.2

Hardeman W, Johnston M & Johnston DW et al. 2002, 'Application of the theory of planned behaviour in behaviour change interventions: a systematic review', *Psychology and Health*, vol. 17, no. 2, pp. 123–158.

Montano DE & Kasprzyk D 2008, 'The theory of reasoned action, theory of planned behaviour and the integrated behavioral model', in K Glanz, BK Rimer & K Viswanath (Eds), *Health behavior and health education: theory, research and practice*, 4th edn, Jossey-Bass, San Francisco, CA.

Further reading 2.4

Bandura A 1997, *Self-efficacy and the exercise of control*, WH Freeman, New York, NY.

Bandura A 1986, *Social foundations of thought and action: a social cognitive theory*, Prentice Hall, Englewood Cliffs, NJ.

McAlistair AL, Perry CL & Parcel G 2008, 'How individuals, environments and health behaviour interact: social cognitive theory', in K Glanz, BK Rimer & K Viswanath (Eds), *Health behavior and health education: theory, research and practice*, 4th edn, Jossey-Bass, San Francisco, CA.

3

Theories on change in communities and communal action for health

Many of the factors that influence health and health-related behaviour can be traced to social structures and the social environment, the local community in which people live. For these reasons, understanding social structures and how to engage and mobilise local communities is important in contemporary health promotion practice.

In the past, the 'community' has been seen simply as a collection of individuals or a 'venue' through which it is possible to reach large numbers of people to bring about larger scale health behaviour changes than might be typical through more individual forms of intervention. Many early community-based programs such as the Stanford Heart Programmes in the 1970s could be characterised this way. However, in contemporary health promotion practice, communities are viewed as dynamic systems with inherent strengths and capabilities that can be influenced and supported in ways which will improve health. This chapter consider three theories for working with communities:

- the diffusion of innovation theory, which entails introducing new ideas into communities;
- community organisation, which involves key approaches by organisations and workers to bring about change in local communities; and
- community building, whereby communities are made more central in decisions about their futures.

3.1   Diffusion of innovation theory

The systematic study of the ways in which new ideas are adopted by communities has its roots in the examination of the ways in which new agricultural technologies were introduced into both developed and developing countries. Over time these studies have been expanded to the introduction of new ideas, practices and technologies in other disciplines, including health. The most widely acknowledged researcher of the diffusion process in relation to health innovation is Everett Rogers who synthesised experience from hundreds of case studies to develop the theory of innovation diffusion and applied it to a wide variety of settings.

Diffusion is defined as 'the process by which an innovation is communicated through certain channels over time among members of a social system' (Rogers 2003). An innovation is defined as 'an idea, practice or object perceived as new by an individual' (ibid). In this case, it is important to emphasise the *perceived* newness of an idea, regardless of its first use or discovery. If an idea is new to an individual, then it is an innovation.

Diffusion of innovation theory has evolved through examination of the processes by which innovations are communicated and adopted (or not). The work of Rogers and others has identified five general factors that influence the success and speed with which new ideas are adopted in communities. Understanding of these factors is central to the application of diffusion theory to health promotion innovations. The factors are:

- the characteristics of the potential adopters;
- the rate of adoption;
- the nature of the social system;
- the characteristics of the innovation; and
- the characteristics of change agents.

Some individuals and groups in society tend to be quicker to pick up new ideas than others, while others tend to be more suspicious of change and slow to respond. Stereotypically, farmers are cautious in their response to innovation and younger people are faster to adopt new ideas.

Rogers used a system of classifying different adopters into categories according to the time it takes for adoption to occur.

- **Innovators** are those 2 to 3 per cent of the population who are quickest to adopt new ideas. However, they may be regarded as fickle and are less likely to be trusted by the majority in the community.
- **Early adopters** are those 10 to 15 per cent of the population who may be more mainstream within the community, but are the most amenable to change and have some of the personal, social or financial resources to adopt the innovation.
- The **early majority** are those 30 to 35 per cent of the population who are amenable to change, and have become persuaded of the benefits of adopting the innovation.
- The **late majority** are those 30 to 35 per cent of the population who are sceptics and are reluctant to adopt new ideas until such time as the benefits have been clearly established.

■ The **laggards** are the final 10 to 20 per cent of the population who are seen to be the most conservative, and in many cases actively resistant to the introduction of new ideas.

As indicated by the different percentages for each group, Rogers suggested that their distribution in a population matches the 'normal' probability distribution curve.

From this simple classification it is possible to see how age, disposable income and exposure to the media are, for example, all important variables which will define the different types of adopter and influence the speed of uptake of innovations. As ever, it is essential to know the community with whom you are working and what is likely to influence their response to new ideas.

Rogers also showed that the cumulative number of adopters can be plotted against time to produce the S-shaped curve shown in Figure 4 below. He emphasised that different innovations take vastly different time periods to introduce to the majority of the target population and, in some cases, will never reach the entire population. The increasing difficulty of influencing late adopters and the residual group of laggards translates into diminishing returns on effort in health programs, and this needs to be recognised in their planning and evaluation.

What becomes obvious from an examination of Roger's theory is the importance of identifying ways of speeding up the adoption process. Factors in different social systems greatly influence the rate of adoption of new ideas. For example, 'traditional' communities, such as rural communities, where the population is more homogenous and inward looking, will generally take

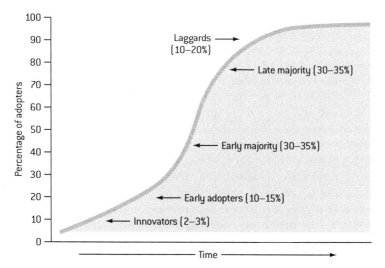

Figure 4 S-shaped curve of diffusion of innovations in communities

longer to adopt any innovation, partly because their exposure to innovations is less common and they may have evolved to be more suspicious of change. In other social groups, change and innovation are much more common, particularly in societies with well-developed communication systems. As a consequence these populations are more experienced in dealing with innovation and better equipped to support the process of diffusion.

An analysis of programs has led to the identification of characteristics of innovations consistently associated with successful adoption. If we consider as an example what is involved in supporting changes in food choices in a population, these characteristics would include:

- compatibility with prevailing socioeconomic and cultural values of the adopter. For example, if a change in diet is being advocated in a particular community, it is more likely to be adopted if the food is based on traditional food sources;
- clarity of the relative advantage of the innovation compared with current practices, including perceived cost effectiveness, as well as usefulness, convenience and prestige. Is the food (such as fresh fruit and vegetables) conveniently available at a price that people can afford?;
- the simplicity and flexibility of the innovation. Those that require simple actions and can be adapted, modified or 'reinvented' to fit different circumstances are more likely to be successful. Is the food simple to prepare and consume, requiring no new cooking methods? Can the preparation and consumption of healthier foods be adapted to established local patterns?;
- the reversibility and perceived risk of adoption. Innovations perceived as high risk or involving an irreversible change in practice are less likely to be adopted. Whether the food will involve the use of new cooking equipment that would have to be purchased, for example; and
- observability of the results of adopting an innovation to others who may be contemplating change. For example, stories in local news sources show the impact of a changed diet on a person's life.

Although it is rare for any innovation to meet all of these criteria, an understanding of these characteristics can help in the development of programs as well as in the identification of implementation problems. For example, in trying to influence the diet of Aboriginal communities in remote parts of Australia it has been very important to recognise that the promotion of more fresh food in the diet assumes that there are ways of buying, storing and cooking fresh foods; this may involve more preparation time than other methods; and may require significant changes in existing food consumption patterns. Not surprisingly, change has been hard to introduce into these communities.

Finally, Rogers identifies the importance of the 'change agent' who facilitates the adoption of change in a population. This may be an independent person working with a community to introduce an innovation or a person from the community who is operating to facilitate change. Allied to this, community members can act as role models for other adopters. A selection of appropriate role models, particularly from among community leaders, can help accelerate the rate of adoption in a community.

There is a clear coincidence of ideas between Rogers' studies of the diffusion process and Bandura's social change theory. The latter emphasises the central role of social modelling in learning about innovation and providing motivation for its adoption.

Diffusion theory is not only applicable to the introduction of new ideas into communities, but can also be considered in relation to organisations where the 'adopters' may be employees or professional groups and the change agents may be managers and professional leaders. This is of great importance in the context of health promotion, both in terms of creating supportive environments for health and in the long-term maintenance of programs. The same type of analysis as that described above can be applied to organisations. Many studies have examined, for example, the introduction of innovations to service organisations, particularly in healthcare settings (see Greenhalgh et al. 2008).

Commentary

Diffusion of innovation theory has been developed and tested in a wide variety of settings and for many different purposes. It provides an excellent diagnostic tool for analysing how and why populations respond to the introduction of new ideas, emphasising the importance of systematic research and planning to maximise the chances of success. The coincidence of themes with social cognitive theory further emphasises the importance of role modelling and the reinforcement of change through social support.

Diffusion theory is of particular importance in guiding programs that are devoted to maximising the adoption of projects which have previously been shown to be effective and is a critical tool in the transfer of evidence-based practice. However, there are limitations to the theory especially in relation to the concept of laggards. It may not only be conservative attitudes and resistance to change that prevent them from adopting new behaviours, but also a lack of resources or other structural barriers. An uncritical adoption of diffusion theory may lead to 'victim blaming' of those least able to adapt to change and may reinforce inequalities that are not necessarily due to individual choice.

3.2   Community organisation and community building

Working with local communities or communities of interest (such as gay groups, indigenous and ethnic minority groups, or groups representing people with disabilities) has been a central strategy for health promotion workers to improve health or address specific problems. Community organisation has been defined as 'the process by which community groups are helped to identify common problems or goals, mobilise resources, and in other ways develop and implement strategies for reaching the goals they have collectively set' (Minkler 1990).

At the community level, several strategies for community organisation have evolved over many years. The most widely recognised typology to describe these approaches was developed by Rothman (in 1968) who identified three models of practice: locality development, social planning and social action.

- **Locality development** emphasises community participation and methods that promote ownership of issues. This approach to community mobilisation is strongly process-oriented, focusing on consensus, cooperation and building community capacity to define and solve community problems. In this model the role of a professional practitioner is as a catalyst and facilitator rather than a leader.

- By contrast, **social planning** is more task-oriented and expert-driven. It is based on a rational–empirical approach to problem definition, and involves professional 'planners' in the development of solutions. The role of the practitioner in this model is one of 'fact gatherer and analyst' and program implementer. This model reflects epidemiological analysis of health problems, and a tightly organised, professionally determined, planned programmatic response.

- The third model, **social action**, is characterised by both a concern for processes which build community capacity and with the achievement of tangible change in a community in favour of the most disadvantaged. Achieving such change inevitably involves shifts in power relationships and resources. The practitioner role in such a model is one of advocate and mediator on behalf of disadvantaged groups.

In proposing these models, Rothman made it clear that none of the models is mutually exclusive, but rather that efforts at community mobilisation will tend towards one or another of the three categorisations. The use of the term 'locality development' has been criticised because it implies that this model of community organisation is applicable only to geographically defined communities. The alternative and the more commonly used term is 'community development'.

Community organisation conceived of in these ways is a useful way of linking individuals, community groups, workers and leaders in a community. It provides a framework within which interventions can be planned and implemented at several levels. For example, developing a program to reduce childhood injury in a community may involve a mix of locality development (working with local community groups to share ideas on the nature of the problem and discussion of possible solutions), social planning (introduction of traffic calming devices into the local environment), and social action (local advocacy for safe pedestrian crossings).

Theories and models of community development continue to evolve, in part in reaction to the perceived limitations of Rothman's typology. Key criticisms concern the extent to which these early models of community organisation were too problem based (seeking solutions to pre-defined problems), and had their roots in approaches to development that were significantly dependent upon outside technical expertise and professional support. These approaches fail to capture the importance of building capacity within communities and, related to this, to foster community empowerment.

At the heart of the distinction between Rothman's construct of community organisation and what Minkler refers to as 'community building' are concepts of empowerment and capacity building. Empowerment is defined by Minkler (1998) as 'a social action process in which individuals, communities and organisations gain mastery over their lives in the context of changing their social and political environment to improve equity and quality of life'. Minkler and others argue that empowerment becomes a fundamental resource that can be used in a variety of situations to improve opportunities for health.

Rissel (1994) has proposed an empowerment 'continuum' that helps to differentiate between stages in the development of empowerment. In this model the stages can apply equally to individuals and communities.

- Health professionals can work with people in ways that increase an individual's confidence that they have the capacity to act in ways that will bring about change;
- Involvement in mutual support groups, self-help or action groups builds and expands social networks and provides opportunities for further personal development. During this process an individual may become critically aware of the wider social forces that are acting on them and their community. Participation in and the influence of community groups is important in both psychological and community empowerment. It is often how people learn new skills that they may be able to use in other situations and also builds the capacity of communities to solve problems.
- As the community becomes more empowered it will work on specific issues, link with other groups to take wider action and ultimately may engage in collective political or social action.

Goodman et al. (2002) define community capacity as 'the characteristics of communities that affect their ability to identify, mobilise and address social and public health problems'. They help to develop our understanding of the multiple dimensions of community capacity. For example, they see community capacity reflected in the number and skills of local leaders to take up issues, the levels of trust and willingness to work together within communities and the ability of local communities to freely share information and to solve problems in innovative and effective ways. They also point out that the capacity of communities is built up over time and so it is important to understand the history of the community and how this has shaped its current circumstances.

Bush, Dower and Mutch (2002) have further developed the dimensions of community capacity and developed a way of identifying and monitoring community capacity. This can assist health promotion practitioners working with local communities to identify current levels of capacity and to identify ways in which community capacity can be further developed. They stress the importance of building capacity to address particular issues or needs—it is something that needs to be developed by 'doing'. They have identified four broad domains of community capacity:

- **network partnerships**—these are the relationships between groups and organisations within a community or network. This includes both the comprehensiveness and the quality of the relationships, that is, are all of the significant groups and organisations involved and what is the nature of their involvement;
- **knowledge transfer**—the development, exchange and use of information within and between the groups and organisations within a network or community;
- **problem solving**—the ability of the groups and organisations within the network or community and of the network or community itself to use well-recognised methods to identify and solve problems that arise in the development and implementation of an activity or program;
- **infrastructure**—refers to the level of investment in a network by the groups and organisations making up the network. This includes both tangible and non-tangible investments, such as investment in policy and protocol development, social capital, human capital and financial capital.

Bush and his colleagues developed their framework based on an extensive review of the literature and case studies. They believe that a key component of building capacity is also building sustainability. Increases in community capacity that are also accompanied by increases in infrastructure are seen as being most sustainable.

When thinking about working in and with communities it is important that practitioners reflect on the extent to which their work is focused on problems that have been identified by the community or by people or services outside the community. For example, service providers may decide that the biggest issue in a community is domestic violence while the community itself may be more concerned with the high levels of crime in the area. Negotiating these different perspectives will be important in planning effective action. It is also important to reflect on whether there is a problem- (or deficit) or strengths-based approach to an issue. For example, the focus of the action may be on high levels of obesity in a community or on the development of improved recreational facilities.

Figure 5 below shows how health promotion practitioners can have an important role in different types of initiatives. In general, those approaches that are based on an assessment of community needs, engage and empower communities, and contribute to increased community capacity, are most likely to achieve sustainable, long-term outcomes.

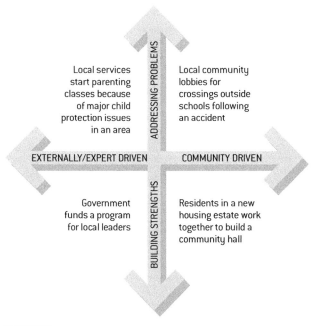

Figure 5 Dimensions of community organisation and capacity building

The complexity of community-based action and the 'shared' control has meant that demonstrating outcomes from community organisation and development is very difficult. As growing evidence of the important role of the social determinants of health in creating opportunities for health has emerged in the past decade, there is greater interest by both practitioners and policy makers in working at the community level to create health-supportive environments. In order to attract the level of resources required to bring about sustained change, clear and convincing arguments to justify use of limited health resources in community settings are required. Often these programs do not have a direct health focus that will lead to short-term health outcomes. In developing its *Guide to Community Preventive Services*, the US Task Force on Community Preventive Services developed a model that makes clear the intermediate outcomes we might expect from community-based activity and the community resources and values that are important to consider in shaping the program (Anderson et al. 2003). It is these middle-level (intermediate) outcomes (refer to Figure 6 below) rather than long-term changes in self-reported health and other health or social indicators that are often most important in documenting changes in community capacity and empowerment (see Minkler, Wallerstein & Wilson 2008).

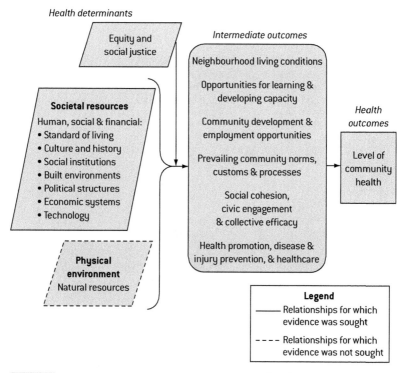

Figure 6 Centres for Disease Control and Prevention (CDC) community guide

Commentary
Unlike the theories and models of health behaviour change at the individual level, community organisation does not lend itself so comfortably to highly structured study and comprehensive theory development. It is not easy to plan or control. Increasingly health promotion practice will involve working

with local communities to create health supportive environments. The lack of a strong public health evidence base for this work means that it is important to develop projects that have a clear, logical pathway that justifies investment of health resources over long periods of time. We should also develop skill in using the extensive evidence bases of other disciplines (such as sociology, demography and political science) to guide and expand our theoretical base.

Community organisation approaches as described by Rothman and others provide a practical framework through which health promotion workers can think about ways in which they may work most effectively with geographically defined communities, or with communities of interest. There is a growing body of literature that reports on the evaluation of complex, community-based interventions. Over time, this will improve our ability to account for the high variation in context (time, place, issue, person) that influences the course and effectiveness of community interventions.

Community organisation approaches enable health promotion workers to address the underlying social determinants of health. It encourages the involvement of communities in defining the problems that they face and in taking action to address them, and enhances the likelihood that changes brought about within communities can be sustained.

Although empowerment of individuals, groups and communities is implied in community organisation approaches it is not necessary for local people to define the problem to be addressed or to take major responsibility for action. Several critics feel that community organisation models often take a 'deficit' approach to thinking about communities—focusing only on problems rather than community strengths. As a consequence, such approaches may fail to recognise and build on the existing strengths in communities.

Despite these perceived limitations there are many examples of situations when the use of the community organisation framework will provide practical guidance on how health promotion workers can work with local communities and service providers to tackle significant health problems.

Community-building based on empowerment is conceptually attractive, but difficult to deliver in practice. Empowerment of individuals and communities is a time-intensive process, one that requires a high level of trust and commitment between those involved and a willingness by the health promotion worker to relinquish power. This is especially challenging when working with the most disenfranchised and marginalised groups in society.

Despite a high level of interest in concepts of community building, community capacity, and the related concept of social capital, these are approaches that also have limitations. For example, there is a risk that focusing on the need to build community capacity may indirectly pass responsibility to communities to solve their own problems, regardless of the root causes. There is an underlying assumption that the most important social forces impacting on people can all be changed at a local level. This will not always be the case. In addition, by working with the most visible leaders in local communities, health promotion workers can further empower the empowered and continue to marginalise those who are disenfranchised.

3.3 Summary

This overview of approaches to working in and with communities to improve health demonstrates the breadth of action that is characteristic of current health promotion thinking. This ranges from approaches that are strongly based on building community competency and control as an integral element to achieving improvements in health, through to those which are overtly health-goal directed and which draw on a sophisticated understanding of how to speed the diffusion of pre-designated ideas in communities.

The diffusion of innovation theory provides guidance on how to introduce new health practices or services into a community. The framework of community organisation described by Rothman provides a sound foundation for working with local communities. Both help health promotion workers to define what it is they are intending to achieve and provides practical guidance on how this can be done. They help us to think about why, how and in what way local communities may be involved in health promotion programs.

The (re)emergence of empowerment and capacity building as drivers in community development reminds us of the importance of seeing communities and their individual members as having strengths and capacities that need to be recognised and developed. Each of these approaches has to be considered on its merits, and placed in the context (people, place and time) in which a program is being developed. Several themes can be drawn from this overview.

- The diffusion of new ideas and practices through communities does not occur by chance, and can be significantly influenced by effective change agents in communities. The importance of effective mass communication and role modelling is emphasised in this process.
- A focus on working at the community level has the advantage of dealing more overtly with the social, economic and environmental determinants of health that have their origins in local conditions.

- It provides opportunities for empowering individuals and communities to take action that will improve their health.
- Skills for health include not only those required to take personal actions that will protect and support health but also the ability and capacity to act collectively.
- Reducing health inequalities in health may involve investing additional resources in building the capacity of those communities that are most disadvantaged to actively participate in and guide programs to improve their health.

References

Anderson LM, Scrimshaw SC, Fullilove MT, Fielding JE & the Task Force on Community Preventive Services 2003, 'The *Community Guide*'s model for linking the social environment to health', *American Journal of Preventive Medicine*, vol. 24, no. 3s, pp. 12-20.

Bush R, Dower J & Mutch A 2002, *Community capacity index*, Centre for Primary Health Care, University of Queensland, Brisbane. Available online at http://www.uq.edu.au/health/docs/2009/CCI.pdf.

Goodman RM et al. 1999, 'Identifying and defining dimensions of community capacity to provide a basis for measurement', *Health Education and Behaviour*, vol. 25, no. 3, pp. 258-278.

Greenhalgh P, Robert G & Bate P et al. 2008, *Diffusion of innovation in health service organisations*, John Wiley and Sons, London.

Minkler M (Ed.) 1998, *Community organizing and community building for health*, Rutgers University Press, Gaithersburg, MD, p. 40.

Minkler M 1990, 'Improving health through community organisation', in K Glanz, BK Rimer & K Viswanath (Eds), *Health behavior and health education: theory, research and practice* Jossey-Boss, San Francisco, CA.

Minkler M, Wallerstein N & Wilson N 2008, 'Improving health through community organisation and community building', in K Glanz, BK Rimer & K Viswanath (Eds), *Health behavior and health education: theory, research and practice*, 4th edn, Jossey-Bass, San Francisco, CA.

Rissel C 1994, 'Empowerment: the holy grail of health promotion', *Health Promotion International*, vol. 9, no. 1, pp. 39–47.

Rothman J 2001, 'Approaches to community interventions', in J Rothman, JL Erlich & JE Tropman (Eds), *Strategies of community interventions*, Peacock Publishers, Itascam Ill.

Rogers EM 2003, *Diffusion of innovations*, 5th edn, Free Press, New York.

Further reading 3.1

Oldenberg B & Glanz K 2008, 'Diffusion of innovations', in K Glanz,
BK Rimer & K Viswanath (Eds), *Health behavior and health education:
theory, research and practice*, 4th edn, Jossey-Bass, San Francisco, CA.

Rogers EM 2002, 'Diffusion of preventive interventions', *Addictive Behaviours*,
vol. 27, pp. 989–993.

Further reading 3.2

Minkler M (Ed.) 2004, *Community organising and community building
for health*, Rutgers University Press, NJ.

4

Models which guide communication to bring about behaviour change

As has been outlined in the previous chapters, effective health promotion strategies are best developed by engaging individuals and communities in the issue to be addressed. This involves understanding the beliefs and knowledge that people have about a problem and their skills in addressing it, as well as broader community understanding of why the issue is important and how it can most effectively be tackled.

Clear communication between health promotion practitioners and those they are trying to influence is essential. Several concepts and models of how this can best be done have emerged, and three of these are outlined below.

4.1 Health literacy

In the past decade, health literacy has emerged as a concept that can help to shape the content and delivery of health education. Low literacy (poor reading and writing skills) is associated both directly and indirectly with a range of poor health outcomes. People with poor literacy skills are less responsive to health education, less likely to use disease prevention services, and are less successful in self-management of disease. The effects of poor literacy can be mitigated through adaptations to health education content and methods that take account of the needs of those with poor literacy. In past decades considerable effort has been made to reduce the complexity and density of written materials, and to use alternative forms of health communication that are not so reliant on the written word.

Growing awareness of the relationship between literacy and health has prompted closer examination of theories of literacy and their potential application in guiding health education. Literacy is generally acknowledged as having two distinctive elements—those that are task-based and those that are skills-based. Task-based literacy focuses on the extent to which a person can perform key literacy tasks such as read a basic text and write a simple statement. Skills-based literacy focuses on the knowledge and skills an adult must possess in order to perform these tasks. These skills range from basic, word-level skills (such as recognising words), to higher level skills (such as drawing appropriate inferences from continuous text). From these basic elements different 'types' of literacy can be identified ranging from the literacy skills needed to be able to function effectively in everyday situations (functional), to more advanced cognitive and literacy skills which can be used to actively participate in everyday activities and to apply new information to changing circumstances (interactive), through to the most advanced cognitive skills which can be applied to critically analyse information, and to use this information to exert greater control over life events and situations (critical literacy). These skills can be developed through formal education and through informal personal experiences.

To better understand health literacy as a distinct concept, it is helpful to recognise that literacy is both content and context specific. Even individuals with higher levels of general literacy (task and skills-based), may not be able to consistently apply their knowledge and skills in situations requiring specific content knowledge, or in unfamiliar contexts—such as in relation to health knowledge, or a healthcare environment. The concept of health literacy can be seen as emerging from a growing awareness of content specific literacy in a health context.

The World Health Organization (WHO) has defined health literacy as 'the cognitive and social skills which determine the motivation and ability of individuals to gain access to, understand and use information in ways which promote and maintain good health' (1998). This definition signals that health literacy comprises a set of skills that enables individuals to exert a higher degree of control over the personal and social determinants of health.

Using insights from the broader study of literacy, health literacy can also be categorised into different levels of functional, interactive and critical health literacy. These different levels progressively reflect greater autonomy and personal empowerment in decision-making, as well as engagement in a wider range of health actions that extend from personal behaviours to social action to address the determinants of health. Progression between types is not only dependent upon cognitive development, but also exposure to different forms of communication and message content.

Conceptualising health literacy in this way has important implications for the content and methods of health education and health communication. In content, health education should not only be directed at changing personal lifestyle or improving compliance with prescribed disease management strategies. It can also be used to raise awareness of the social determinants of health, and be directed towards the promotion of personal and social actions that lead to modification of these determinants. In methods, health educators are challenged to communicate in ways that draw upon personal experience, invite interaction, participation and critical analysis. Such an approach to education and communication draws on established principles in adult education and community development that can be applied equally to people with low and high levels of basic literacy.

Figure 7 below provides a summary of the concept of health literacy as an outcome to health education. It is based on recognition of prior knowledge and capability (1), leading to tailored health education and communication (2). It shows the purpose of the health education as being directed towards the development of relevant personal knowledge and capability (3), and interpersonal and social skills (4, 5). Health literacy is the *outcome* of health education and communication rather than a factor that may influence the outcome (6). Figure 7 indicates that people who have better developed health literacy will thus have skills and capabilities that enable them to engage in a range of health enhancing actions including modifying personal behaviours (7), as well as social actions for health and influencing others towards healthy decisions such as quitting smoking, or engaging in social action for health (8, 9). The results are not only improved health outcomes but also a wider range of options and opportunities for health (10).

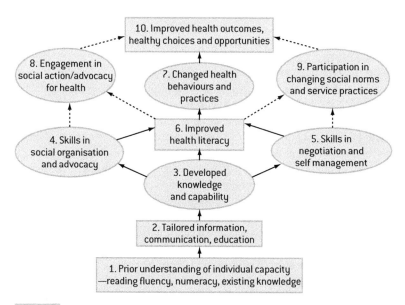

Figure 7 Developing interactive and critical health literacy skills

Case study: antenatal education

Researchers in Sydney used the health literacy concept to examine antenatal education and to make recommendations on how the concept might be applied to improve the educational program (Renkert & Nutbeam 2001). They found that antenatal education was often provided in a very structured form in group classes for pregnant women and their partners, with a goal of achieving compliance with a highly prescribed set of predetermined behaviours relating to childbirth.

Using the concept of health literacy, antenatal educators identified an alternative approach to the organisation and delivery of the program. Following the structure in Figure 7 on page 39, such a program would begin by assessing variation in underlying literacy and language skills at the commencement of the program and tailoring it to better match the existing literacy skills of participants. It would support the highest possible level of participation in the learning process, and through the educational processes, develop the competence and confidence of participants to obtain and evaluate information from a variety of sources, and the skills and confidence to act on that information—focusing on the development of functional and interactive health literacy skills. The goal of the modified program would be to develop in women the ability to 'access, understand and use information' in ways that enable constructive interactions with healthcare providers, and support critical, independent application of new knowledge to 'promote and maintain their health and that of their children' (ibid).

Commentary

Health literacy is an emerging concept that prompts wider thinking on the content and methods used in health education, balancing an established focus on health behaviour change with the potential of health education as a tool that enables action on the social determinants of health. Improving health literacy in a population involves more than the transmission of health information, although that remains a fundamental task. Helping people to develop confidence to act on that knowledge and the ability to work with and support others will best be achieved through more personal forms of communication, and through community-based educational outreach. If theories such as social cognitive theory help us to understand better the process of achieving change, the concept of health literacy emphasises the importance of using a broader repertoire of content and methods of communication in health education. Use of the concept highlights the potential of education to strengthen political action, and to ensure that the content of health communications not only focuses on personal health, but also on the social determinants of health. However, the measurement of health literacy remains undeveloped, and the concept has not yet been fully tested as a basis for intervention through systematic research. Care needs to be taken in the application of the model, lest the advocacy exceeds the evidence for its adoption.

4.2 Communication–behaviour change model

The communication–behaviour change model was developed by McGuire (in 1981) to design and guide public education campaigns. It is included in this chapter because the model is based on communication 'inputs' and 'outputs' which are designed to influence attitudes and behaviour in similar ways to the theories and models described in earlier chapters. The five communication inputs described by McGuire are:

- The **source**—the person, group or organisation from whom a message is perceived to have come. The source can influence the credibility, clarity and relevance of a message. For example, the same message delivered by a government source, a celebrity or a non-government organisation will have different credibility and relevance to different target audiences.
- The **message**—what is said and how it is said. The content and form of a message can influence audience response. For example, the use of fear or humour to communicate the same message may provoke different responses from different target audiences. Practical considerations such as the length of the message, its form, and the complexity of the language and tone of 'voice' used also need to be considered.
- The **channel**—the medium through which a message is delivered. Traditional media includes television, radio and print (e.g. newspapers, pamphlets, posters), as well as techniques such as direct mail. More recently, information technology has opened up a range of new media for use in communicating health messages, including the internet (e.g. dedicated health information websites and informal social networking sites) and mobile phone text messages. Issues to be considered in selecting a channel for communication include its potential reach, the cost of use and differences in the complexity of message which can be communicated.
- The **receiver**—the intended target audience. Recognising differences in audience segments and their media preferences is of importance for matching the right message to the right channel from the right source. Social and demographic variables such as gender, age, ethnic background, literacy level and location, as well as current attitudes, behaviours and media access can all be considered as a part of this input.

- The **destination**—the desired outcome to the communication. This may include the acquisition of new knowledge, a change in attitudes or the confidence to act, as well as more specific behavioural changes.

The communication–behaviour change model can be very useful in conceptualising and designing mass communication strategies. For example, in trying to highlight a men's health issue such as the risk of prostate cancer, it will be important for the source of the message to be someone respected by the men most at risk and with whom they can identify. The message itself will need to be conveyed in an acceptable or agreeable way, such as by using humour, and through media used by men. Decisions will also need to be made about which messages can best be communicated by the various media. A good understanding of the target population will help to determine the subgroups requiring dedicated targeting (e.g. those of high or low literacy, ethnic minorities, etc.), as well as greater specificity in the intended outcome (e.g. general awareness raising or predefined behavioural outcomes such as attendance for screening).

This model also provides a 12-step sequence of events, representing outputs from a communication, which link initial exposure to a message to a long-term change in behaviour. The 12 steps are:

- exposure
- attention
- interest
- understanding
- skill acquisition
- attitude change
- memorisation
- recall
- decision-making
- behaviour change
- reinforcement
- maintenance.

According to the model, for a communication strategy to be effective the message has to be carefully designed and delivered through an appropriate channel to reach the target audience. The population has to be exposed to the message (no mean feat in itself!), pay attention to it and understand it. Even if a message has achieved this, there are still eight more steps to the achievement of sustainable health behaviour change.

Once understood by an individual, the message must create an inclination to change, which will be reflected in an attitude change that is stored and maintained until such time as the receiver is in a position to act on his or her attitude change. Once the decision to change has been made and acted on, the new behaviour will need reinforcement in order to be maintained.

These inputs and outputs can be put together as a matrix to illustrate the need to change the input mix depending on the targeted output. Different sources, messages and channels will be required to reach different receivers and achieve different outcomes.

Commentary

Even though this model is not based on substantial empirical testing in the way that some other models have been developed (e.g. the health belief model, the theory of reasoned action), it is based on the same structure of relationships between beliefs and perceptions, and attitudes and behaviour, that are illustrated by these other models.

The communication–behaviour change model shows just how difficult it can be to develop a public communication campaign which, by itself, leads to sustainable behaviour change. This model provides an excellent overview of the range of issues that need to be considered in the development of a public education campaign. Although several major public intervention programs have been based on this model (such as the first Stanford three-cities program in the US, which was intended to reduce the risks for heart disease in the community), progressive experience using the mass media for public communication has led to a better understanding of the advantages and limitations of media campaigns in terms of cost, reach and effect. Media campaigns are now more commonly used to influence public knowledge, attitudes and opinions as a part of a more comprehensive strategy that places mass communication within a wider repertoire of interventions.

4.3   Social marketing

Social marketing evolved as a technique to influence social norms and health behaviours in the 1970s. These early approaches were based on the simple adaptation of established commercial marketing techniques for the achievement of social change. There are several competing definitions of social marketing, but one of the simplest and clearest was provided by Andreasen (1995), as follows:

> Social marketing is the application of commercial marketing technologies to the analysis, planning, execution and evaluation of programs designed to influence the voluntary behaviour of target audiences in order to improve their personal welfare and that of society.

This definition of social marketing relates to the use of marketing techniques to influence behaviour for individual or social benefit.

Social marketing has become very popular as a technique in health promotion for the simple reason that funding agencies find it relatively easy to understand and invest in. As a consequence, significant public health funding in developed and developing countries alike has been devoted to social marketing and related health communication. Fortunately, there is reasonable evidence from a 2006 review that carefully managed social marketing programs can be effective in improving diet, increasing exercise and tackling substance misuse in a range of target populations. In social marketing, a marketing organisation will use its resources to:

■ understand the perceived interests of target market members;
■ enhance and deliver benefits associated with a product, service or idea; and
■ reduce barriers that interfere with the adoption or maintenance of that product, service or idea.

Target market members, in turn, expend their resources (such as money, time or effort) in exchange for the offer when it provides clear advantages over alternative behaviours. Success of a social marketing program is defined primarily in terms of its contribution to the wellbeing of target market members or to society as a whole. This definition emphasises the importance of a benefit to individuals and society. It is this benefit and the nature of the relationship between the 'buyer' (target market) and 'seller' (health organisation or practitioner) that helps to distinguish social marketing for health promotion and disease prevention from that of commercial marketing.

In commerce, marketing is designed to influence consumer choice. The marketplace exchange is the commodity or service sold and money collected. Success can be measured in the volume of these exchanges. Although improving product knowledge or changing attitudes and values towards a product may be a means to influence purchasing behaviour, these are not in themselves the objective of marketing.

Social marketing is likewise intended to influence how people think and, ultimately, how they behave. Similarly, it is based on a change in behaviour with costs and benefits to the individuals concerned. For example, immunisation offers protection against measles; a parent considers the costs and benefits of this 'product', and decides whether or not to engage in this behaviour— essentially whether to 'buy' immunisation. The success of an immunisation program can be consequently measured in the number of people who are immunised.

Although costs may not be financial and the benefit not material, the same objective of achieving a change in behaviour is at the heart of the social marketing process. However, social marketing does differ from commercial marketing in its intent to benefit the target population and/or society in general, rather than only to benefit the marketer. Thus the *relationship* between the 'seller' and 'buyer' will in many cases be very different from that in commercial marketing. The definition above emphasises that this is a voluntary exchange, based on mutual fulfilment of self-interest—both parties are clearly seen to benefit, rather than one exploiting the other.

The social marketing wheel

The social marketing wheel was originally developed by Novelli (in 1984) and proposes six sequential stages to a social marketing strategy. These stages account for the needs of the target audience, the development and implementation of a marketing strategy to reflect those needs and a tracking of audience response to the strategy.

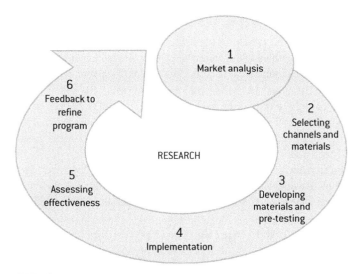

Figure 8 Social marketing wheel

Marketing analysis

Social marketing has a strong 'consumer' orientation rather than a focus on selling a product or service through persuasive communication. This requires a good understanding of the priority population through market research into underlying knowledge of and attitudes to the issue or service and potential channels for communication (e.g. literacy, media use). Such market research is intended to lead to clearly defined marketing objectives and strategies for achieving them, and to allow for segmentation of different priority populations with different needs and interests. This is followed by development and testing of the marketing plan elements and subsequent implementation; for example, finding the groups of people that have low immunisation rates and exploring the reasons why some children have not been immunised.

Selecting channels and materials: the marketing mix

Marketing strategies are multifactorial and generally based on achieving a balanced mix of four major inputs, commonly referred to as the four Ps— product, price, promotion and placement.

The product is often difficult to define in a health promotion program; we are not often selling tangible goods or services, or immediate rewards for expenditure. Identifying what is 'on offer' and presenting an appropriate image for the priority population is essential. For example, in the case of immunising children it is important to distinguish between the procedure (the injection), the service offered (the visit to the GP or nurse) and the health status achieved (protection against future disease), as each may have different meaning and relevance to different target populations.

The price signifies the relationship between the costs and benefits of the 'product'—the return on investment. The costs may be real or perceived and include financial (e.g. the cost of visiting the GP), social (e.g. social pressure from the family to have the child immunised) or opportunity costs (e.g. taking time off work to attend a local clinic). Equally, the benefits may be real or perceived. The costs and benefits of advocated actions need to be carefully considered in relation to different population subgroups. In the case of immunisation, many parents may never have seen a child with a vaccine-preventable disease and have no real conception of what it is they are trying to prevent. Strategies to effectively communicate benefit, and reduce costs (real and perceived) have to be developed. Such an analysis is similar to the analysis of benefits and barriers described in the health belief model.

A wide range of techniques for promotion are used in social marketing. These include the purchased media (e.g. advertising, leaflets), non-purchased media (e.g. news coverage), sponsorship, participation events, direct selling, competitions and so on. Selecting the most appropriate channel, message delivery and source for the priority population is essential for success. Such an analysis could be based on the development of 'inputs' described by McGuire in his communication–behaviour change model.

In all forms of marketing the final step to success is in finding high access points for a defined priority population, that is, the right placement. This critical aspect of 'access' has often been neglected in the development of health programs. For example, the use of health screening services is determined in part by the convenience of access and the sensitivity of service providers to language barriers and different cultural and religious norms.

Achieving the right marketing mix is at the heart of the social marketing process. Failure to address any one of the four elements will reduce the chances of success, as will over-concentration on one element alone. There can be nothing more frustrating than, for example, mounting a successful campaign to promote uptake of immunisation, only to find that service providers are unable to cope with increased demands for services and stocks of vaccine running low.

Implementation, assessment and feedback

These stages represent the management of a social marketing program and are not unique to social marketing in that sense. Monitoring the implementation of a program according to a planned schedule and monitoring its impact and effects according to predetermined objectives are routine elements to all health promotion programs. Social marketing is an iterative process, and the model is intended to account for changes in audience responses and the external environment governing the implementation process (e.g. funding and organisational structures). In this final stage, any changes to the environment are considered alongside information from the evaluation to guide the evolution of the next cycle.

Commentary

Social marketing offers a sophisticated model for achieving defined behavioural objectives in identified priority populations. It is less a theory in the formal sense defined earlier than a planning model for health promotion. The social marketing wheel illustrates the cyclical nature of the marketing process, offering a systematic, research-based process for problem solving which includes the planning, implementation and feedback loops common to such models. It offers an opportunity to integrate elements of different theories (such as the health belief model and the communication–behaviour change model), using each to advantage in a complete program model.

It is particularly useful because it encourages creative approaches to the analysis of issues and the development of programs, especially in relation to the development of channels for communication and messages. For example, social marketing has encouraged us to look outside typical analyses of populations (e.g. age, gender, social class) in order to define consumer groups based on their media consumption or family structure. Social marketing has supported experimentation with the use of a wide repertoire of different intervention methods, including mass communication and the sponsorship of events and competitions, all of which have been effectively used for health promotion. Social marketing also supports a strong consumer focus in the development and delivery of programs.

It would be a mistake, however, to imagine that social marketing simply involves taking marketing strategies from the commercial sector and applying them to achieve health goals. The 'product' in terms of improved health or protection against disease is often intangible; the 'price' usually not financial. Health promotion programs also operate from a different philosophical and moral base to many traditional marketing campaigns which are driven by financial gain. In such circumstances the marketing techniques to achieve sustained mass behaviour change are a great deal more complex than promoting a tangible product based on financial exchange in the commercial marketplace.

4.4 Summary

Each of the concepts and models presented in this chapter provide insight and guidance on the strengths and weaknesses of education and communication for health promotion. The social marketing theory provides a substantial model for planning and executing an integrated campaign that places more traditional health education and communication in a wider context.

Each model illustrates in different ways the limits of different forms of mass communication in producing substantial mass behaviour change, and also demonstrates the potential of well-structured and organised communication strategies in raising awareness of health issues, securing public and political support for different forms of health promotion intervention, and in supporting related personal and community action.

The communication–behaviour change model and social marketing both indicate the complexity of mass communication and illustrate:

■ the importance of adequate market research to define issues, segment target populations and test communication ideas;

■ the need to match the source, message, medium and receiver in developing mass communication campaigns;

■ the need to consider a wide range of different methods of communication and different venues and settings (promotion and placement) in the development of mass communication campaigns; and

■ the importance of basing the evaluation of mass communication campaigns on realistically defined outcomes.

The health literacy concept provides a bridge between these practical techniques for health communication and the broader empowerment goals of health promotion. It places emphasis on health education methods and content that:

■ support more interactive forms of communication which draw upon personal experience and invite participation in the learning process and a critical analysis of health issues; and

■ improve people's knowledge, understanding and capacity to act not only in relation to individual health behaviours but also on the social determinants of health.

References

Andreasen, AR 1995, *Marketing social change: changing behavior to promote health, social development, and the environment*, Jossey-Bass, San Francisco, CA.

Renkert S & Nutbeam D 2001, 'Opportunities to improve maternal health literacy through antenatal education', *Health Promotion International*, vol. 16, no. 4, pp. 381–388.

World Health Organization (WHO) 1998, *Health promotion glossary*, WHO, Geneva. Available online at http://www.who.int/healthpromotion/conferences/7gchp/track2/en/index.html.

Further reading 4.1

Institute of Medicine 2004, *Health literacy: a prescription to end confusion*, National Academies Press, Washington DC.

Nutbeam D 2008, 'The evolving concept of health literacy', *Social Science and Medicine*, vol. 67, pp. 272–278.

Pignone M, DeWalt D & Sheridan S et al. 2005, 'Interventions to improve health outcomes for patients with low literacy', *Journal of General Internal Medicine*, vol. 20, no. 2, pp. 185–192.

Further reading 4.2

Hornick Robert C (Ed.) 2002, *Public health communication: evidence for behavior change*, Erlbaum Associates, Mahwah NJ.

Maibach E & Parrott RL (Eds) 1995, *Designing health messages: approaches from communication theory and public health practice*, Sage, Thousand Oaks, CA.

McGuire WJ 2001, 'Input and output variables currently promising for constructing persuasive communications', in RE Rice & C Atkin (Eds), *Public communication campaigns*, 3rd edn, Sage, Thousand Oaks, CA.

Further reading 4.3

Andreasen AR 2006, *Social marketing in the 21st century*, Sage, Thousand Oaks, CA.

Gordon R, McDermott L, Stead M & Angus K 2006, 'The effectiveness of social marketing interventions: what's the evidence?', *Public Health*, vol. 120, pp. 1133–1139.

Storey JD, Saffitz GB & Rimon JG 2008, 'Social marketing', in K Glanz, BK Rimer & K Viswanath (Eds), *Health behavior and health education: theory, research and practice*, 4th edn, Jossey-Bass, San Francisco, CA.

5

Models for change in organisations and creation of supportive organisational practices

Goodman et al. (2002) have succinctly described the problems and potential rewards of facilitating change in organisations, as follows:

> Organisations are layered. Their strata range from the surrounding environment at the broadest level, to the overall organisational structure, to the management within, to work groups, to each individual member. Change may be influenced at each of these strata, and health promotion strategies that are directed at several layers simultaneously may be most durable in producing the desired results. The health professional who understands the ecology of organisations and who can apply appropriate strategies has a powerful tool for change.

Health promotion practitioners are interested in influencing organisations for a number of reasons.

■ We are usually employed by organisations and have an interest in ensuring that our own organisation is able to support the work that we are doing.

■ We are interested in influencing the activities or policies of other organisations that have an influence on the health of the population.

■ We have to find ways to enable organisations to work together to promote the health of the population.

Unlike many of the theories and models described in previous chapters, the application of existing theories concerning organisational change is far less developed and analysed, or systematically tested. In this chapter we look at models of how organisational change can be applied to organisations and models that describe and explain how organisations can work together, often referred to as intersectoral action.

5.1   Theories of organisational change

Most of our understanding of how to produce organisational change has come from the development of management theory (and practice). This body of theory and knowledge has developed to explain organisational change for a variety of purposes, often in relation to improving organisational performance. It provides useful clues as to how to analyse different organisational settings and how to plan for change. Often these theories identify a number of stages or phases of change within organisations.

Goodman et al. (2002) propose a four-stage model for organisational change that is applicable to health promotion practice. They emphasise the importance of recognising the different stages and matching strategies to promote change in each of the stages. These stages, presented below, are similar in structure to the stages of change theory and the diffusion of innovation theory discussed in previous chapters.

- Stage 1—**awareness raising**. This stage is intended to stimulate interest and support for organisational change at a senior level by clarifying health-related problems in the organisational environment and identifying potential solutions. For example, awareness raising may involve senior managers and administrators in the education system becoming concerned about tobacco control and recognising the potential role to be played by the education system. These 'senior level administrators' are likely to be the most influential in decisions to adopt new policies and programs in an organisation. If they are convinced of the importance of a problem and the need for a solution involving their organisation, then the strategy moves to the next stage.

- Stage 2—**adoption**. This stage involves planning for and the adoption of a policy, program or other innovation that addresses the problem identified in Stage 1. This includes the identification of resources necessary for implementation. In larger organisations, this stage will often involve a different level in the management structure—the 'gatekeepers'—who are more closely associated with the day-to-day running of an organisation. In the example above this could involve school principals and senior teachers responsible for school curricula and organisation. Ideally, this stage will involve negotiation and adaptation of intervention ideas in order to make them compatible with the circumstances of individual organisations. This element of adaptation is often essential to the adoption of change in organisations, but frequently missed by those attempting to disseminate new ideas through organisations.

- Stage 3—**implementation**. This stage is concerned with technical aspects of program delivery, including the provision of training and material support needed for the introduction of change. Using the same example, this could involve classroom teachers, as they will be most directly responsible for the introduction of change. This stage may involve training and the provision of resource support to foster the successful introduction of a program. This 'capacity building' is essential for the successful introduction and maintenance of change in organisations. Many policy initiatives fail at this point because too little attention is given to the detail of the implementation process and too little support is offered to the individuals at the level at which implementation takes place in an organisation.

- Stage 4—**institutionalisation**. This stage is concerned with the long-term maintenance of an innovation once it has been successfully introduced. Senior administrators again become the leading players by establishing systems for monitoring and quality control, including continued investment in resources and training.

In developing their ideas, Goodman et al. have drawn upon several established theories that describe and explain organisational change and development. These theories have evolved to include environmental influences and how the norms and values of entire organisations are transformed. The related concepts of organisational climate and culture and organisational capacity need to be recognised and understood in the execution of a staged approach to organisational change described above.

Organisational climate is often referred to as the 'personality' of organisations, meaning those characteristics that distinguish one organisation from another, based on the collective perceptions of those who live and work in a particular environment, and that influence their behaviour. For example, some schools are more or less authoritarian in their relations with students; public services are more or less customer focused; some work sites value and reward staff loyalty more than others. These characteristics are seen as dynamic and are affected by a wide range of variables, many of which are external to the organisation. The term 'organisational culture' is often used interchangeably with climate, but is distinguished as meaning a set of values and assumptions about an organisation that have formed over time and are more stable and resistant to change. Both organisational climate and culture can influence an organisation's capacity to function effectively, and in turn may determine the outcome of efforts to bring about change in organisations. 'Organisational capacity' can also be seen in more practical terms, such as having appropriately trained personnel, effective management systems and sufficient resources. Organisational climate, culture and capacity are all important variables that will influence the pace and extent of change which may be achieved through the four-stage process described above.

Achieving organisational change may involve interventions designed to alter the organisational climate and build organisational capacity. This capacity building is an important element of effective health promotion practice. Hawe et al. (1997) have defined capacity building as:

> the development of sustainable skills, structures, resources and commitment to health improvement … to prolong and multiply health gains many times over.

Capacity building is sometimes described as the invisible work of health promotion. It has been described as including activities as diverse as canvassing the opportunities for a program, lobbying for support, developing skills, supporting policy development, negotiating with management, partnership development and organisational planning.

Commentary

The model developed by Goodman et al. is particularly helpful in illustrating the ways in which organisations function at different levels, how the achievement of organisational change may be achieved in a staged process, and how each stage may require involvement of different levels in an organisation. The model is most useful in situations where an organisation is viewed as a potential host institution to previously developed health programs. It does not so easily accommodate health promotion strategies that seek to help organisations to develop in a more holistic way, such as to develop organisational policy and practices as a means to creating safe and health supportive environments for workers and clients.

5.2 Models of intersectoral action

As well as working with organisations as potential host institutions for existing programs, and as a means to creating supportive environments for health, we need increasingly to work with organisations as partners in the development and implementation of health promotion programs. This process is often referred to as 'intersectoral action'. WHO (1997) defines intersectoral action for health as:

> a recognized relationship between part or parts of the health sector with part or parts of other sectors which has been formed to take action on an issue to achieve a health outcome … in a way that is more effective, efficient or sustainable than could be achieved by the health sector working alone.

There are few theories or models that define this process and none that enjoy universal recognition among health promotion workers, but there have been several recent attempts to review experience in intersectoral action and related activities such as coalition building and partnerships. These reviews have identified different forms of intersectoral action and sets of factors that are important to understanding the process by which organisations, or parts of organisations, work together.

Glendinning et al. (2002) have identified that two of the most fundamental factors influencing the nature and success of intersectoral working are the extent of dependence and trust between partner organisations. Put simply, if one organisation depends upon cooperation with another to achieve its goals, and there exists a high level of trust between them, then joint action is more feasible and more likely to be successful. By working together organisations may be able to ensure that their services are more relevant and coordinated, and they have access to sufficient resources to make a difference.

For example, food suppliers may be willing to work with the health sector to improve the supply of fresh fruit and vegetables to a specific area. The food suppliers would do so with the intention of increasing sales of these foods (their core business); the health sector will do so to improve nutrition in a population (their core business). As partners they are to some extent codependent: each able to fulfil their core business more successfully by working together rather than in isolation.

Trust between organisations is also crucial to the development of strong intersectoral partnerships. Trust is developed over time and is built on relationships between individuals and their organisations. For this reason many successful partnerships are between individuals and organisations that have worked successfully together in the past. The relationships that have developed are based on respect for all those involved and recognition of each party's unique capacity to contribute to achieving shared goals. Building trust can be very challenging. In many relationships between organisations there is an imbalance in control over resources and capacity to influence decision-making. There may also be a history of competition or antagonism. In such cases it becomes essential that the relationship and the benefits to all those involved are transparent and fair.

Although we often speak of partnerships or coalitions, it is important to remember that there is no one model of the way in which organisations work together. At the one end of the spectrum, the relationships between organisations may be simply one of sharing information and meeting regularly to discuss common problems. At the other end of the spectrum, partnerships can be highly structured, where roles, responsibilities and outcomes are mandated.

As illustrated in Figure 9 opposite, the continuum between networks, alliances, partnerships, coalitions and highly structured collaborations often reflects increased formal agreements between organisations to work together in certain areas and a greater investment in organisational resources.

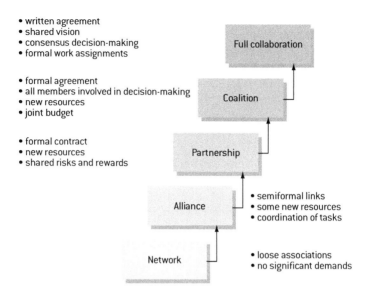

• written agreement
• shared vision
• consensus decision-making
• formal work assignments

Full collaboration

• formal agreement
• all members involved in decision-making
• new resources
• joint budget

Coalition

• formal contract
• new resources
• shared risks and rewards

Partnership

Alliance

• semiformal links
• some new resources
• coordination of tasks

Network

• loose associations
• no significant demands

Figure 9 Continuum of ways organisations work together

Beyond these basic factors of codependence and trust, a review of intersectoral action in Australia has proposed a framework for understanding the factors that will influence effective intersectoral action. In this model six factors were identified as important dimensions to effective intersectoral action:

■ the **necessity** for the sectors or organisations to work together;
■ the **factors** that are providing the opportunity for them to work together;
■ the **capacity** to work together;
■ established **relationships** that will allow them to achieve their goal;
■ the action they are undertaking should be **planned** and able to be evaluated; and
■ the action should be **sustainable**.

Understanding the context

Successful collaboration between organisations is built on the foundations of necessity and opportunity. Organisations are more likely to be open to collaboration and change if it helps them to pursue core business more effectively or efficiently. This core business may have nothing to do with health in a direct sense, but may have an indirect impact on health; for example, if the core business is transport or housing programs, or the activities of private sector companies promoting different foods. In addition to achieving their organisational goals, organisations are also interested in working together to:

- attract or protect resources;
- protect or gain in their areas of influence; and
- be seen as good corporate citizens.

Understanding the strength of the motivation for organisations to work together assists in understanding the level of commitment they will be willing to make and the risk they will be willing to take.

The opportunity for taking action is reflected in immediate organisational priorities. These may be in response to crises within organisations or a response to unpredicted events outside the organisation. For example, a number of fatal football injuries may make it more likely that sporting organisations will be receptive to advice concerning changes in rules recommended by the health sector. However, without the infrastructure to undertake action, such opportunities to work with other organisations to achieve common goals may be missed.

Assessing the infrastructure

Many of the factors that contribute to either the success or failure of a particular activity are seen as related to the capacity of the organisations to undertake that activity. This capacity is primarily reflected in:

- the level of organisational support for the activity (including compatible structures and decision-making processes);
- adequate levels of resources (including time, financial resources and infrastructure); and
- a skilled workforce.

The other crucial aspect of infrastructure is the relationship that exists between the organisations involved. These relationships are generally a mix of formal and informal links, and provide the mechanism within which actions can be developed and conflicts resolved. Without adequate infrastructure it can be difficult for organisations to sustain action over time or adapt to changing circumstances.

A planned approach to action and sustainability

Building and sustaining relationships between sectors towards common goals is a difficult task. Many of the conditions for success (or failure) are in place long before any specific action is taken, and it is important to not only plan the details of the project but also to account for the context in which it is being undertaken and the ability of the infrastructure of the organisations to deliver. From reviews of practice, several issues have emerged as important in the implementation of a project that requires cooperation between different agencies:

- a clear recognition of why it is important for the organisations to work together, including agreement on how the issue and the solution are defined and what role they see for their respective organisations in the implementation process;

■ acknowledgment that the process is emergent and changing;

■ the need for flexibility in negotiation over roles and responsibilities;

■ a definition of a clearly articulated and achievable goal that is understood and valued by the different organisations involved in a project;

■ an agreement on a way of working—this may mean working on small, well-defined tasks initially to build trust and confidence in a working relationship before seeking to implement more significant changes;

■ opportunities for renegotiation, including identification of the length of time to which organisations are committed and allowing for redefinition of tasks, roles and relationships;

■ a commitment to joint ownership—any sense that one partner is imposing on another invariably leads to resistance and damage to the relationship; and

■ the allocation of resources—staff, space, money, information and administrative support.

The case studies in Table 4 below illustrate how such a comprehensive analysis can help us understand why some activities are successful and others difficult.

Table 4 Application of the model for understanding intersectoral action

Case study: the Children's Services Health & Safety Committee	Case study: access to children's services
Background	*Background*
Following an outbreak of measles in 1991, the Health & Safety Committee was formed to improve health and safety policies and practices in childcare centres. Major service providers, unions, training bodies, public health units and academics have been able to work together effectively on this issue.	The same core group of people and organisations that successfully established the Health & Safety Committee have had much more difficulty in addressing lack of access to children's services for children whose parents are on low incomes and not in the workforce.
Necessity	*Necessity*
It was clear at all levels of the childcare and health sectors that they needed to work together to improve policies and practices.	There is not a high level of concern in either the healthcare or childcare sectors about this issue, and the ways in which both sectors could work together is not clear.

(Continued)

Table 4 (*Continued*)

Case study: the Children's Services Health & Safety Committee	Case study: access to children's services
Opportunity	*Opportunity*
The dramatic increase in the number of children in care in the past decade and concern for the children's health supported the action. The measles epidemic and growing epidemiological evidence of the risks associated with care provided strong triggers for action.	Current community concern about the provision of children's services is focused on the needs of working parents. There are few triggers for action, no obvious policies to support action in this area, limited data on the nature and extent of the problem, and no new ways of thinking about the issue.
Capacity	*Capacity*
Although specific resources for the committee were limited there was a high level of organisational support by all involved (including a research grant) and skilled workers to undertake any action.	The organisations and individuals involved are already stretched and, although there are high levels of organisational support, there are few resources for taking action.
Relationship	*Relationship*
Most of the organisations involved had worked together before in some way. Because the action did not require high levels of joint planning or resource allocation the relation-ships were able to be loose and flexible.	New relationships will need to be formed to bring together all the stakeholders in this issue. There is little time to identify, contact and build support.
Action	*Action*
Over the past two years the committee has focused on research into current policies and practices and the development of model policies.	Because there is little understanding of the nature and extent of the problem and little history of working together, there is no clear plan of possible action. In this case, few of the conditions for effective action are in place. Rather than invest time in developing a plan of action it would be better to look at ways of making the necessity for the action more apparent, to create an environment where action is seen as important, and to look at ways of increasing the capacity of the organisations to take action.
Sustainable outcomes	
It is now important for the committee to look at ways in which it can sustain any gains they have made. This will involve more formal recognition of the committee by both sectors and the allocation of specific resources.	

Commentary

As many of the most entrenched health problems we face, especially those related to addressing health inequality, have their roots in the wider social system it is inevitable that health promotion workers will continue to need to work across organisations to improve health. For these reasons, the concepts and values that underpin notions of collaboration and partnership have resonance with many health promotion workers. They sit easily with a recognition that action to improve health is not only the responsibility of the health system, but also that of many other organisations. This has led to a high level of investment in partnership working, coalition building and the types of intersectoral action described above.

However, there is increasing concern that the level of investment required in establishing and maintaining effective relationships may be greater than the benefits. For this reason it is important to develop a critical approach to deciding if and how these relationships should be developed and what it is that we hope will be achieved by them.

Although there is not a single agreed model or theory of intersectoral action, there is now a strong body of experience that provides some guidance on those factors important in effective action. There is also a better understanding that the relationships between organisations can take many forms and it is not always essential to establish highly formalised relationships if the organisational goals of all those involved can be met through more informal means.

Additionally, it is clear that if organisations are to work effectively together they often need to change internally in order for them to have the capacity to work with other organisations; for example, they may need to change their funding cycle or processes for making decisions. In particular they may need to employ staff who are able to work effectively across organisations. In the literature these people are often referred to as 'reticulists' or 'organisational spanners'.

5.3 Summary

Although the models described above are not strictly theories according to the criteria described at the beginning of this guide, they are based on systematic observation and analysis of organisational change, and do offer guidance on factors influencing the successful introduction and maintenance of change in organisational settings. Further, systematic testing of these ideas in planned programs will be necessary to clarify their usefulness and identify further refinements. These models provide useful guidance on the different steps required to introduce and sustain a program in different organisational settings. In particular they highlight:

- the need to understand the core business of an organisation and its organisational structure, determine how a health promotion program can fit within these parameters, and help achieve core business;
- the need to work with individuals at different levels in an organisation as well as between organisations;
- the inherently 'political' nature of the task of influencing senior managers;
- the importance of flexibility in negotiation with 'gatekeepers' concerning the adoption of a program;
- the need to support those individuals responsible for the delivery of a program or innovation; and
- the need to establish a system for long-term maintenance and quality control.

One of the major reasons the health sector is interested in working with other organisational structures is to bring about systematic and lasting change that will address some of the basic determinants of health, for example, safe workplaces, improved living conditions or the development of recreational facilities. Understanding how to do this most effectively has the potential to have profound impacts on health.

References

Glendinning C, Powell M & Rummery K (Eds) 2002, *Partnerships, new labour and the governance of welfare*, Policy Press, Bristol.

Goodman RM, Steckler A & Kegler MC 2002, 'Mobilizing organisations for health enhancement: theories of organisational change', in K Glanz, BK Rimer & K Viswanath (Eds), *Health behavior and health education: theory, research and practice*, Jossey-Bass, San Francisco, CA.

Hawe P, Noort M, King L & Jorden C 1997, 'Multiplying health gains: the critical role of capacity building in health promotion programs', *Health Policy*, 39, pp. 29–42.

World Health Organization (WHO) 1997, *WHO International Conference on Intersectoral Action for Health*, WHO, Geneva. Available online at http://whqlibdoc.who.int/hq/1997/WHO_PPE_PAC_97.6.pdf.

Further reading 5.1

Butterfoss FD, Kegler MC & Francisco VT 2008, 'Mobilizing organizations for health promotion: theories of organizational change', in K Glanz, BK Rimer & K Viswanath (Eds), *Health behavior and health education: theory, research and practice*, 4th edn, Jossey-Bass, San Francisco, CA.

Further reading 5.2

Butterfoss FD, Goodman R & Wandersman A 1993, 'Community coalitions for prevention and health promotion', *Health Education Research*, vol. 8, no. 3, pp. 315–330.

Butterfoss FD, Kegler MC & Francisco VT 2008, 'Mobilizing organizations for health promotion: theories of organizational change', in K Glanz, BK Rimer & K Viswanath (Eds), *Health behavior and health education: theory, research and practice*, 4th edn, Jossey-Bass, San Francisco, CA.

Harris E, Wise M & Hawe P et al. 1995, *Working together: intersectoral action for health*, Australian Government Publishing Service, Canberra.

O'Neill M, Lemieux V & Groleau G et al. 1997, 'Coalition theory as a framework for understanding and implementing intersectoral health-related interventions', *Health Promotion International*, vol. 12, no. 1, pp. 79–85.

6

Models for development and implementation of healthy public policy

Public policy has been simply described as 'what governments decide to do or not to do' (Dye 1972). It involves the decision to act on a particular problem, and then includes subsequent decisions relating to implementation and enforcement (Walt 1994). Through the process of developing policy, governments decide which problems or issues are important enough to warrant government attention.

Public policy making is a political activity—a process in which a range of participants with different agendas and concerns from both inside and outside government compete to put issues on the policy agenda and to formulate policy. They interact in a variety of ways. Policy making involves deliberation among individuals, communities and organisations on solutions for public problems, each contributing their own perspective and evidence. There is often debate about values, ideas and priorities. Finally, policy making involves participants engaging in decision-making—either reaching a consensus or marshalling a majority of votes. Research-derived evidence of 'what works' is only one component of public policy making and implementation.

Engaging effectively in developing and implementing public policy is an increasingly important role for those involved in health promotion. This chapter defines healthy public policy, describes the stages in the policy cycle and presents models for influencing public policy, contributing to evidence-based policy making and guiding policy implementation.

This chapter examines three different models and frameworks that help us to better understand the policy development process and how to influence it.

6.1   What is healthy public policy?

Not all public policy has an impact on health, and policies that do may have a positive or negative impact. Understanding the impact of all types of policy on health has been an important part of contemporary health promotion, and has led to the development of the concept of 'healthy public policy'. Kickbusch (2004) described healthy public policy as policy that:

> … makes healthy choices possible or easier for citizens. All government sectors (including agriculture, trade, treasury, education, housing, transport and communications, for example) have roles in the creation and implementation of public policy and all should be accountable for the health and equity consequences of their policy decisions.

To engage effectively in the policy process we need to have the knowledge and skills to communicate effectively with governments, contribute to framing problems and solutions, and influence decisions about which of these is selected to become a government's policy response. We also need to be able to monitor and influence implementation and ensure that there are mechanisms in place to assess and report on intended and unintended effects of policy on health. This is a developing area of health promotion practice.

6.2 A framework for making healthy public policy

Nancy Milio (1984) developed a conceptual framework explaining how successful policies to improve health are developed. In this framework, policies are seen as passing through the following discrete (albeit overlapping) stages during their development—initiation, formulation, adoption, implementation, evaluation and reformulation. These stages are part of a continuous social and political process that is not, in practice, linear—nor, necessarily, rational. In this framework, four groups usually make up the participants in policy formulation and implementation:

- policy makers (usually politicians and public servants);
- policy influencers (who can be groups inside and outside of government, sometimes known as policy communities);
- the public (audiences, consumers, taxpayers and voters), whose opinion ultimately affects the adoption and implementation of policy; and
- the media (print and electronic) that influence both policy makers' and the public's understanding of, and attitude towards, an issue and/or proposed solutions.

Although the formulation of public policy often appears to be driven by an influential individual or group, Milio (and others) argue that it is the organisations they represent and not the individuals themselves that should be the focus when analysing their interests and resource bases.

The formulation of a specific policy draws together organisations and groups that may share the policy goal, but have different responsibilities with regard to the content and final decision-making. They may have diverse or competing interests in relation to the policy content, the processes through which the policy is formulated and the ways it is implemented. For example, government is ultimately the policy maker in relation to gun regulation, while the policy influencers may be the police, gun lobbies, public health agencies or community coalitions attempting to influence content, process of formulation and implementation.

In this framework, the public is not considered to be a policy maker or a policy influencer, other than through formally organised bodies. Instead, the views of the public on an issue are considered to be part of the 'climate' within which policy making is occurring. If it is to be possible to influence the formulation of a particular public policy, identifying and assessing the following is necessary:

- the social, economic and political context within which action is being proposed (the social climate);
- the parties with mandated responsibility for the formulation of policy on this issue;
- the interests of those who wish to influence policy formulation— what they hope to win or lose and where they are willing to compromise; and
- the capacity of the organisations or groups wishing to formulate or influence policy to put in place strategies that will allow them to represent their interests successfully.

With any policy issue there are multiple perspectives on the problem, its causes or determinants, and the solutions that should be reflected in the public policy response. Taking the deaths and injuries from shootings as an example, for some groups the problem is seen as being uncontrolled access to guns; for others it is people who use guns irresponsibly or illegally. In Australia over the course of a decade, several tragic mass shootings dramatically shifted the social climate regarding solutions to shooting-related deaths and injuries from a concern for the 'rights' of gun owners towards a concern for broader community interests to be protected from the consequences of uncontrolled access to guns.

In this case, the groups that had used evidence of the positive impact of tighter gun control on deaths and injuries from shooting to advocate for tighter gun control found that their power to influence change increased over the decade. The change in social climate combined with effective advocacy for tighter gun control as a response meant that the policy influencers were better placed to put forward tough proposals for gun control in the belief that government would be unlikely to ignore broad-based public support. The policy influencers who were opposed to gun control searched for ways to re-exert their influence and put forward arguments to the government to counterbalance community sentiments. Where these latter groups had succeeded at the beginning of the decade in removing gun control from the public policy agenda, by the end of the decade overwhelming public support for gun control saw it re-introduced to the policy agenda and ultimately, to legislation, implementation and enforcement.

This example illustrates how influencing the formulation of public policy requires the use of effective public and interpersonal communication strategies to create a social climate to support change. This, in turn, requires the use of research-derived information (where it is available) to inform, persuade and motivate a variety of audiences, including the public. In the gun control example, leadership on the issue was provided by credible spokespersons who informed policy makers, policy influencers and the public about the relationship between uncontrolled gun ownership and gun-related deaths and injuries, effective responses and the benefits for the wider population of tough gun control policy. The leaders also challenged the arguments and evidence used by opponents.

Commentary

Milio's framework identifies four groups who have major roles in the formulation of public policy—policy makers, policy influencers, the public and the media. Knowing and understanding who these groups are and what their interests or purposes are will highlight the multiple points of potential influence for those of us wanting to affect the formulation of public policy to create conditions for health and equity.

6.3   Evidence-based policy making to promote health

For a long time a major reason given for the lack of healthy public policy was that there was a lack of scientific evidence regarding 'what to do' to address specific public health problems. In recent years, however, there has been a burgeoning of evidence to guide policy makers seeking to formulate policy to intervene effectively to promote and protect health, to prevent disease and injury and, on some occasions, to increase equity in health. But epidemiologists and other population health researchers still claim that it is difficult to have their findings taken up by policy makers; while policy makers claim that it is difficult to find relevant evidence upon which to base policy.

In the real-life course of policy formulation, different evidence is used by the four policy groups (see Milio's framework above) for a variety of purposes—to describe and frame problems, to identify solutions, and to select from among these the ones that should or will be adopted into policy and implemented.

The relationship between research-derived evidence and policy is a growing field of research in its own right. Carol Weiss (1979) developed a set of models that explain different ways in which evidence can be used in policy formulation.

- In the **knowledge-driven model**, the emergence of new knowledge from research automatically creates pressure for its application in policy, and the transfer of new knowledge into policy is relatively quick. An example from public health is the development of a new vaccine that leads to public pressure for its immediate adoption, even when an analysis of benefit relative to cost indicates that there may be alternative investments that could produce greater public health benefits.

- In the **problem-solving model**, evidence derived from a variety of sources is gathered and synthesised as a starting point for policy formulation. The implication is that evidence is the primary driver of decisions about what 'solutions' a policy is proposing. This model implies that policy making is a rational, iterative, linear process with a clear beginning and end. There are few examples of the application of this model in public health practice.

- In the **interactive model**, research knowledge is utilised as one source of evidence in the decision-making process, to be considered alongside evidence derived from experience, political insight and social pressures. The policy outcome is achieved following negotiation among policy makers and policy influencers.

- In the **political model**, evidence is used to justify a predetermined position, based on the values and beliefs of policy makers. It relies on the selective inclusion and interpretation of data. The exclusive use of mass media campaigns and school-based interventions to address complex problems such as drug misuse or antisocial behaviour are examples of this model.

- In the **tactical model**, research-derived evidence is used to delay a decision or to avoid responsibility for an unpopular decision. In this model the normal uncertainty of research findings is exploited as a mechanism for delaying a decision until 'more evidence is gathered'. Alternatively, where an unpopular decision is made, evidence may be used to justify that decision, even if the evidence is rather weak.

Although it is tempting to believe that public policy is the outcome of rational consideration of research-derived knowledge by neutral, rational people or organisations, in reality this is rarely the case (Bowen, Zwi 2005). It is much more likely that the interactive, political and tactical models describe ways that research-derived evidence is used in policy formulation.

As mentioned in the introduction, policy making is inherently political—a process through which diverse and, often, conflicting values and perspectives on issues and solutions, on costs and benefits, and on who will be advantaged and who will be disadvantaged, are negotiated and ultimately decided.

In reality, policy formulation on any particular issue requires a point in time appraisal of:

- what is scientifically plausible (based on current research-derived evidence);
- what is politically acceptable (fits with political values and ideology); and
- what is practical for implementation.

This means that research-derived evidence is most likely to be used in policy formulation if it:

- is currently available and accessible;
- fits with political vision (or can be made to fit); and
- points to actions for which powers and resources are (or could be) available, and the systems, structures and capacity for action exist.

Scientists complain frequently that their research is ignored by policy makers. However, researchers also need to examine whether their choice of subject, method of communication, degree of understanding of the policy-agenda setting, or formulation or implementation processes contribute to their work being ignored.

Evelyn De Leeuw (1993) outlined three determinants of policy making that need to be understood by those interested in creating healthy public policy. These determinants are:

- the bias that stems from the causal, final and normative assumptions and presuppositions of those responsible for policy making and for influencing policy;
- the interest webs of groups seeking to influence policy formulation; and
- the power of organisations to communicate and monitor their intentions.

Assumptions

Policy makers acquire through their professional training and work environments a set of assumptions and beliefs about policy directions that are, then, assumed to apply universally. Three sets of assumptions that affect policy formulation are proposed: those around the relationship between cause and effect; those between intervention and outcome; and underlying values. Together these are seen to form a framework used by policy makers (including influencers, the public and the media) to establish and assess policy objectives, instruments and time frames. Although these assumptions are used to judge the desirability and feasibility of proposed policy options, they are rarely made explicit.

For example, among the people considering policy options to reduce the negative health effects associated with unemployment, these three sets of assumptions appear to influence the views of those involved. The relationship between unemployment (cause) and poor health (effect) is often perceived to be unclear or unproven—are unemployed people more likely to have lost their job because they were sick, or is their poor health the result of unhealthy lifestyle choices rather than unemployment itself? Policy makers (and others) often perceive that a single solution will be sufficient to improve health outcomes, for example, that full employment will solve the problem. And despite the fact that there are fewer jobs available than people to fill them, some policy makers seem to continue to believe that people could find a job if they really wanted to work, despite evidence to the contrary.

Interests

Policy formulation is influenced by the vested interests of each group of stakeholders involved. For example, in efforts to reduce unemployment levels the stakeholders with vested interests include those wanting to deregulate the labour market to promote economic growth, unions interested in ensuring members do not lose their jobs, and welfare groups advocating improved income support for the unemployed.

Although subscribing to the same policy goal (to reduce unemployment), each of these groups needs, primarily, to ensure their own survival and the preservation of their sphere of influence. This may put them in conflict with evidence of what would be the most effective policy to reduce unemployment, and either lead to the removal of the issue from the policy agenda or undermine the effectiveness of the policy option that is adopted. Formulating healthy public policy requires adept analysis to identify overlapping interests and needs, and skilful negotiation to identify acceptable solutions to address these. Providing research-derived information on the health effects of different options may not be sufficient to achieve the desired public policy outcome.

Power positions

The extent to which groups (i.e. policy influencers, the public and the media) are able to influence the framing of problems and solutions, and influence policy formulation and adoption, is closely related to their capacity to identify and understand the strategic intentions of their competitors and allies. For example, if the health sector is seeking to introduce policies to reduce the harmful effects of unemployment on health, it must work with other sectors and organisations. These potential partners may view the health sector's interest in the issue as being a way to get more money to provide health services or as cost-shifting to another sector.

The capacity of organisations (and individuals) to monitor the interests and plans of competitors and allies, and their ability to communicate their own intentions, has proved highly predictive of the success organisations have in influencing policy. For health promotion practitioners it also means ensuring that research-derived evidence (including, but not limited to, epidemiological evidence) must be presented to address stakeholders' interests and concerns, illustrate the likely benefits to them and convey a detailed description of the strategies that will enable them to achieve their own organisational goals.

Commentary

Weiss's models help to identify ways in which to enhance the likelihood that research-derived evidence influences the formulation of public policy. In highlighting the limitations of assuming that policy formulation is a rational, evidence-driven process, she points to the multiple avenues through which evidence can be inserted into the policy process. De Leeuw, on the other hand, offers insight into the characteristics of policy makers (and their organisations) which influence their use of research to guide policy formulation.

6.4   Models for health impact assessment

Health impact assessment (HIA) is a structured process of assessing available evidence to predict the likely impact of proposed policies or programs on the health of defined populations. By undertaking such an assessment it is possible to recommend changes to a policy or program to increase the likelihood of positive health impact and to reduce the likelihood of negative health impact.

The concept of policy impact assessment is now well established, and there are both models and practical examples from environmental, economic and regulatory impact assessments that can be adapted for the purposes of HIA. Some forms of assessment are mandatory in different countries, mostly to determine the likely economic impact and/or impact on quality of life for populations affected by policy change. Few countries or jurisdictions have legislated to make HIA mandatory.

Over the last decade HIA has been applied to a wide range of policy proposals arising from a variety of sectors. A typology that describes the primary drivers of HIA has been developed—legislation (mandated); decision support (voluntary use initiated by policy makers); advocacy (voluntary use initiated by policy influencers); and community empowerment (voluntary use by the public). HIA has also been adapted to enable the specific analysis of the impact of policy proposals on equity. The WHO Commission on the Social Determinants of Health (2008) pointed to the usefulness of this as an approach to identify steps to increase the equity of outcomes likely to result from a proposed policy.

Experience has demonstrated that HIA has particular value in exposing the assumptions and decisions that underlie the formulation of a policy or practice to wider consideration and discussion by the people/populations that are likely to be affected by its implementation. It also exposes the evidence that is available to inform policy decisions and, increasingly, the gaps in the current evidence which need to be addressed by future research. HIA as a method is flexible and adaptable to a variety of circumstances, but is generally based on four core stages—screening, scoping, appraisal and developing recommendations. Each of these stages is discussed below.

Screening: deciding whether to undertake HIA

As HIA is only one way to influence public policy to create conditions for good health, it is necessary to first consider and rule out the utility of other potential approaches before deciding to proceed. A major consideration here is making a judgment on the extent to which the recommendations of an HIA are likely to be valued by the relevant decision makers. If policy makers (or program designers) are reluctant to wait for an assessment or have expressed resistance to potential findings, health promotion practitioners need to consider alternative routes through which to influence public policy.

Scoping: deciding how to undertake the HIA in the available time

Once it has been decided to undertake an HIA, it is necessary to consider how best to do it with the available time and resources. The main concern is ensuring that the HIA can be completed in time to present clear recommendations to policy makers for consideration before any decisions are made. This is one of the most difficult challenges for this methodology as it is essential that political deadlines are met. This means, in some cases, adapting the method to meet the time available.

Appraisal: identifying and examining evidence for potential impacts

This is the core stage of the HIA process and involves:
- identifying the logic framework to map the pathways by which a proposal might be expected to have positive and/or negative effects on the health of a given population; and
- examining the different types of evidence available in order to make a judgment on the potential significance and scale of such impacts.

Issues of particular importance at this stage include:
- identifying the ways a proposal may affect the determinants of health, including socioeconomic factors, environmental conditions, social, community and working contexts, and individual and family lifestyles;

- considering disproportionate impacts of a proposal on different groups within the population in order to expose potential inequity and/or health inequity;
- examining different stakeholder perspectives on a proposal to assess potential impacts. When done well the HIA process can have value in supporting stakeholder engagement with both communities who are likely to be affected and policy makers; and
- incorporating and valuing different sources of evidence, such as that drawn from a mix of disciplines including the physical sciences, biomedicine, psychology, sociology and anthropology. It may also be necessary to generate evidence directly for the HIA, particularly in order to gain the affected communities' perspectives on potential health impacts of a given policy proposal.

Developing recommendations: deciding on what to recommend to the relevant decision makers

Central to this step is understanding the values and requirements of the relevant decision makers in order to increase the likelihood that recommendations from the HIA are adopted. Crucial to framing the recommendations is recognising that decision makers are likely to need to consider the potential of the proposed policy to achieve multiple benefits, of which health is only one. Linking the health benefits to other considerations such as economic development, employment, education and urban regeneration, for example, is likely to enhance an HIA's perceived value.

Review and evaluation

When recommendations have been produced and considered by the relevant decision makers, the purpose of the HIA is essentially complete. However, routine review and evaluation of the contribution of the assessment to policy, practice and, over time, health outcomes (and their distribution) are fundamental steps in best practice. In particular, this stage should assess the extent to which:

- the HIA's recommendations were actually adopted and the reasons why;
- the adopted recommendations had the predicted effects on the determinants of health or the health outcomes;
- those recommendations not adopted had the predicted negative impacts on determinants of health or on health outcomes; and
- there were other unanticipated positive or negative impacts arising from the public policy.

Health in all policies

A variation on the basic concept of HIA has emerged in the concept of Health in All Policies (HiAP) (Stahl et al. 2006). HiAP is an approach that seeks to improve the health of populations both by contributing to the formulation and implementation of healthy public policy using HIA and by highlighting the ways in which the health of populations contributes to the wellbeing and the wealth of nations. In common with HIA, HiAP has its conceptual roots in the environmental and ecological impact analyses that evolved during the 1970s and 80s. In addition, as with health promotion and HIA, HiAP is based on recognition of the interdependence and multidimensionality of policy making; many sectors need to work with others in order to solve the complex problems that must be addressed by societies and our organisations of governance. In practice, the HiAP approach has demonstrated that it is possible to introduce an evidence-based approach to policy making which assesses and discusses the possible health impacts of proposed policy alternatives and to formulate policy that meets the goals of other sectors and is likely to enhance the health of the population.

Commentary

HIA methodologies offer us ways of working effectively across sectors to influence policy formulation and implementation and to create healthy public policy. HIA provides a structured approach to introducing and assessing evidence of the health effects of proposed policy options and to negotiating with policy makers from all engaged sectors on recommendations. A transparent process, HIA clarifies assumptions underlying policy proposals and uses the best available evidence to influence these in the direction of positive health effects. It also offers considerable scope to provide a voice in policy making to individuals and communities most likely to be affected by a new or revised public policy.

Increasingly, HIA is being recognised by policy makers and influencers as a legitimate and useful method to influence public policy formulation, particularly when it necessitates the engagement of multiple sectors. There are increasing initiatives to integrate environmental, social and health impact assessments (as appropriate), drawing on the strengths of each to offer a more sophisticated assessment of public policies attempting to address the multiple causes of many complex problems facing contemporary societies, including, for example, climate change, conflict and poverty.

6.5   Summary

This chapter outlines some of the approaches that can provide us with valuable guidance on ways in which health promotion practitioners, researchers and policy makers can contribute to the generation, formulation and adoption of healthy public policy. Taking the development and implementation of 'healthy public policy' as the goal, the chapter uses Milio's framework to describe four groups of 'actors' engaged in setting policy agendas and formulating public policy. Although it is widely accepted that policy making is not a linear process, a description of a policy cycle nonetheless assists in understanding significant points at which influence may be exerted in policy formulation. Understanding the factors that influence the likelihood of an issue 'making' it onto a government's policy agenda, and those that influence the final decision on which policy option is adopted, can help us to identify potential 'points of influence' for health promotion practitioners. The work of Weiss and others explains how evidence actually influences public policy formulation and helps to demystify the gap between the ideal of evidence-based policy making and the reality. Evidence does not necessarily protect against bias or questionable judgment on the part of policy makers. HIAs offer practical approaches to influencing public policy to become healthy public policy.

Each of these methodologies helps us better understand and work with the reality of policy making, as well as offering opportunities to introduce evidence-based recommendations at different, significant points in the policy cycle to increase the likelihood of positive health impact. Through this we recognise that public policy is not formulated solely based on evidence of the nature and extent of a problem and its causes or determinants. Nor is it formulated entirely based on a single source of evidence of effective strategies to address the problem. It is, rather, the outcome of contested views about each of these things.

In order to understand and influence the process through which a policy is developed, it is necessary to recognise the major stakeholders, their interests, their perceptions of the issue and their preferred solutions. This understanding points to areas of potential conflict and compromise. Although not directly engaged in policy formulation, the public's opinion and the social climate are a vital context that influences policy makers' decisions. Influencing public opinion and the social climate provide further opportunities to shape the likelihood of achieving healthy public policy.

References
Bowen S, Zwi A 2005, 'Pathways to evidence and informed policy and practice: a framework for action', *Public Library of Science Medicine*, vol. 2, no. 7, pp. 0100–0106 (e166).

Commission on the Social Determinants of Health 2008, 'Closing the gap in a generation: health equity through action on the social determinants of health', *Final report of the Commission on the Social Determinants of Health*, World Health Organization, Geneva.

De Leeuw E 1993, 'Health policy, epidemiology and power: the interest web', *Health Promotion International*, vol. 8, no. 1, pp. 49–53.

Dye T 1972, *Understanding public policy*, Prentice-Hall, Englewood Cliffs, NJ, p. 2.

Kickbusch I 2008, 'Adelaide revisited: from healthy public policy to Health in All Policies', *Health Promotion International*, vol. 23, no. 1, pp. 1–4.

Milio N 1987, 'Making healthy public policy: developing the science by learning the art: an ecological framework for policy studies', *Health Promotion*, vol. 2, no. 3, pp. 263–274.

Stahl T, Wismar M, Ollila E, Lahtinen E & Leppo K 2006, 'Health in all policies: prospects and potentials', *Ministry of Social Affairs and Health*, Finland, p. xviii.

Walt G 1998, *Health policy: an introduction to process and power*, Zed Books, London.

Weiss CH 1979, 'The many meanings of research utilisation', *Public Administration Review*, vol. 39, pp. 426–431.

Further reading
Nutbeam D 2004, 'How does evidence influence public health policy? Tackling health inequalities in England', *Health Promotion Journal of Australia*, vol. 14, pp. 154–158.

Further web-based sources of information on HIA
The World Health Organization: http://www.who.int/hia.
The International Association of Impact Assessment has a dedicated HIA section: http://www.iaia.org/sections.
For a practical guide to health impact assessment, see http://www.hiaconnect.edu.au.

conclusion

Theory in practice

This book provides only an introduction to the many different theories and models that have guided health promotion practice. The chapters provide a synthesis of the key elements of the theories and research which have guided their development, and indicate their potential application to practice. Readers who require more detailed information on the different theories should refer to the references and further reading sections at the end of each chapter, or to other more comprehensive publications.

What will be apparent from the content of the different chapters is that the theory guiding practice in health promotion is not yet well developed. The theories concerning psychosocial determinants of health in individuals are the least complex and best tested according to traditional criteria. The different theories and models that may be useful to guide elements of programs directed to community mobilisation, organisational change and policy development are generally less well formed and far less amenable to testing through experimental research designs. However, the importance of community mobilisation and organisational and policy change for health is so great that it is essential to identify and apply our best current understanding of these issues. Research to advance our knowledge and understanding of such processes is of the highest priority in the future.

There is no single theory or model that can adequately guide the development of a comprehensive health promotion program intended to influence the multiple determinants of health in populations. Practitioners need to use local knowledge and experience, and available research information, to make judgments about community needs and the determinants of health that are most amenable to change at any particular time. In developing a comprehensive strategy to tackle a defined health priority, practitioners will be assisted by making judicious use of the theories and models described in this guide. Multilevel interventions will generally be more powerful than single-track programs. Correspondingly, programs may need to be informed by several of the theories and models described in this book in the development of a comprehensive strategy. If applied wisely, these theories will help guide decisions, may predict the likely outcomes and help explain the reasons for success or failure.

Not all practitioners have the position or capacity to operate at multiple levels. In such cases, knowledge of the theories and models in this guide will help practitioners to maximise the potential effectiveness of their interventions and to place into perspective their efforts alongside the range of opportunities for action.

index

References to graphics are shown in *italic* text.